DIET SUPER METABOLISM 2025

110 New Recipes Discover the Secret to an Active and Vibrant Life and Reach Your Weight Goals with the New Frontier of Health

KLARLOCK

DISCLAIMER

This book aims to provide useful and informative material on the topics covered in the publication. It is sold with the understanding that the author and publisher are not engaged in rendering any personal medical, health care, or other professional services in the book. The reader should consult his or her physician, health care provider, or other competent professional before adopting any suggestions in this book or drawing any conclusions. The author and publisher expressly disclaim responsibility for any liability, loss, or risk, personal or otherwise, arising, directly or indirectly, from the use and application of any contents of this book.

NOTE

All the recipes in this book are designed for four people. For this quantity, the ingredients indicated in the recipes must be considered. If you need to change the portion, it is recommended to proportionally adjust the doses of the ingredients. It is also recommended to carefully follow the preparation and cooking instructions to obtain the best result. In the context of this book, when we refer to "a cup" as a unit of measurement for ingredients, we mean using a standard kitchen cup with a capacity of approximately 2 milliliters. It is essential to use a measuring cup to get the right quantities of ingredients. If you don't have a measuring cup, you can use a graduated measuring cup, making sure to correctly correspond to the proportions indicated. Here are some examples 1 Cup of flour 100 gr. 1 cup of rice 200 gr. 1 Cup of Quinoa 200 gr

TABLE OF CONTENT

78 AVOCADO STUFFED WITH TUNA AND LEMON

80 CHERRY TOMATOES STUFFED WITH GOAT'S CHEESE AND PARSLEY

82 BUFFALO MOZZARELLA WITH TOMATOES AND FRESH BASIL

84 RAW VEGETABLES WITH YOGURT SAUCE AND FRESH HERBS

86 QUINOA FRITTERS WITH MIXED VEGETABLES

88 QUINOA SALAD WITH GRILLED CHICKEN

90 WHOLE BREAD CANAPES WITH AVOCADO PESTO

92 LENTIL MEATBALLS WITH YOGURT AND MINT SAUCE

94 MUSHROOM CARPACCIO WITH EXTRA VIRGIN OLIVE OIL AND LEMON

96 CROSTINI WITH CREAM OF WHITE BEANS AND ROSEMARY

98 MIXED BEAN SALAD WITH RED ONION AND PARSLEY

100 COURGET ROLL WITH RICOTTA AND DRIED TOMATOES

102 PUMPKIN SOUP WITH TOASTED PUMPKIN SEEDS

104 BAKED AUBERGINE MEATBALLS WITH TOMATO SAUCE

106 BLACK BEAN SALAD WITH CORN AND PEPPERS

108 GRILLED VEGETABLES WITH AVOCADO AND LIME SAUCE

110 CREAM OF CARROTS WITH GINGER AND CUMIN

112 BRUSCHETTE WITH BEAN BEAN CREAM AND GRATED PECORINO

114 SEAFOOD SALAD WITH TOMATOES AND PARSLEY

116 CROSTINI WITH CHICKPEA CREAM AND CHILI PEPPER

118 BROCCOLI FLAN WITH FRESH CHEESE

120 SWEET AND SOUR VEGETABLES WITH BALSAMIC VINEGAR

122 QUINOA AND CHEESE CROQUETTES

RECIPES FIRST DISHES

171 ZUCCHINI TAGLIATELLE WITH FRESH TOMATO SAUCE

173 PEARL BARLEY WITH ARTICHOKES AND PECORINO

175 ZUCCHINI SPAGHETTI WITH AVOCADO PESTO

177 BROWN RICE WITH ROASTED PEPPERS AND FRESH CHEESE

180 WHOLEWHEAT PENNE WITH CAULIFLOWER AND CRISPY SPECK

182 VENERE RICE WITH GRILLED VEGETABLES AND GREEN OLIVES

184 WHOLE WHOLE RISOTTO WITH ASPARAGUS AND PARMESAN

186 WHOLE WHOLE PASTA WITH AUBERGINES AND DRIED TOMATOES

188 SPELLED SOUP AND SEASONAL VEGETABLES

190 WHOLE WHOLE LINGUINE WITH CLAMS AND TOMATOES

192 WHOLE WHOLE PASTA SALAD WITH TUNA AND OLIVES

RECIPES SECOND DISHES

SIDE DISH RECIPES

280 STEAMED VEGETABLES WITH TAHINI SAUCE

282 ROASTED FENNEL WITH ORANGES AND OLIVES

284 GRILLED AUBERGINES WITH TOMATOES AND MOZZARELLA

286 SAUTEED SPINACH WITH GARLIC AND CHILI

288 STUFFED MUSHROOMS

INTRODUCTION TO THE SUPER METABOLISM DIET

 Welcome to the Super Metabolism Diet 2025, an innovative and scientifically supported approach to optimizing your metabolic health and achieving your ideal weight in a healthy and sustainable way. In an era in which obesity and diseases related to poor nutrition are increasingly widespread, it is essential to adopt effective strategies to improve our metabolism and promote general well-being. But what exactly is metabolism and why is it so important? Metabolism represents the set of biochemical processes that occur within our body to transform the food we eat into energy. It is responsible for regulating body weight, managing blood sugar, and affects our ability to burn calories throughout the day.

An efficient metabolism is essential for maintaining a healthy weight and preventing many chronic diseases. However, metabolism is not a static characteristic of our body; it can be influenced by a number of factors, including our diet, lifestyle, physical activity, stress and sleep quality. The Super Metabolism Diet aims to optimize all of these elements to maximize the efficiency of your metabolism and promote optimal health. This book will guide you through the fundamental principles of the Super Metabolism Diet, giving you a comprehensive overview of the dietary, lifestyle and exercise strategies aimed at boosting your metabolism and achieving your health and fitness goals. We'll explore the science behind metabolism, identify foods that stimulate calorie burning, and discuss best practices for meal planning and preparing nutritious and delicious recipes. Additionally, we'll examine the importance of regular exercise, stress management, and quality sleep to maintain an optimal metabolism and promote overall well-being. Regardless of your current health status or fitness goal, the Diet Super Metabolism can be tailored to your individual needs, allowing you to pursue a personalized path to success. Are you ready to start your journey to a supercharged metabolism and a healthier, more energetic life? Then get ready to transform your body and your health with the Super Metabolism Diet.

WHAT IS THE SUPER METABOLISM DIET

The Super Metabolism Diet is a dietary approach designed to optimize metabolism and promote weight loss in a healthy and sustainable way. It is based on the idea that metabolism can be accelerated through specific food choices, food combinations and well-structured meal regimens. Key features of the Super Metabolism Diet include: 1. Super Metabolic Foods: The diet focuses on incorporating foods that are known to aid metabolism and calorie burning, such as fiber-rich fruits and vegetables, lean proteins, whole grains, and healthy fats. 2. Meal Planning: The diet includes a meal plan that distributes calorie intake in a balanced way throughout the day, with regular meals and snacks to keep the metabolism active.

3. Macronutrient Rotation: A key element of the Super Metabolism Diet is macronutrient rotation, which involves varying carbohydrates, proteins and fats at different meals and days of the week to stimulate metabolism and prevent metabolic adaptation. **4. Exclusion of Processed and Sugary Foods:** The diet encourages avoiding highly processed foods, rich in added sugars and saturated fats, focusing instead on whole, nutritious foods. **5. Adequate Hydration:** Another important component of the Super Metabolism Diet is promoting adequate hydration, encouraging the consumption of water and unsweetened beverages to keep the body hydrated and support metabolism.

6. Physical Exercise: In addition to nutrition, the diet also suggests integrating a regular regime of physical activity to optimize metabolism and promote weight loss. The Super Metabolism Diet aims to improve overall metabolic health by reducing inflammation, stabilizing blood sugar levels and increasing energy. Importantly, the diet does not promote extreme restrictions or unhealthy eating behaviors, but rather emphasizes the importance of making conscious and long-term sustainable food choices.

BENEFITS OF THE DIET

The Super Metabolism Diet offers a number of health and wellness benefits, including: 1. Increased Metabolism: One of the main benefits of the diet is increased metabolism. It promotes greater metabolic efficiency, stimulating caloric combustion and facilitating weight loss. 2. Weight Loss: The Super Metabolism diet is designed to promote weight loss in a healthy and sustainable way. By focusing on nutritious foods and meal planning strategies, it helps reduce excess body fat and improve body composition. 3. Stabilize Blood Sugar Levels: By reducing consumption of added sugars and highly processed foods, the diet helps stabilize blood sugar levels, preventing sudden spikes and drops that can lead to excessive hunger and cravings not healthy.

4. Increased Energy: By combining nutritious foods and maintaining stable blood sugar levels, the Super Metabolism Diet can increase energy levels and improve physical and mental stamina throughout the day. 5. Better Appetite Control: By consuming regular meals and snacks rich in fiber, protein and healthy fats, the diet can help control appetite and reduce excessive cravings, promoting a greater feeling of satiety. 6. Promoting Cardiovascular Health: The reduction in inflammation and stabilization of blood sugar levels associated with the Super Metabolism Diet may help improve cardiovascular health, reducing the risk of heart disease and stroke.

7. Improved Sleep Quality: Adopting a balanced and healthy diet can also positively influence the quality of sleep. By reducing the consumption of foods rich in sugar and caffeine and encouraging proper hydration, the diet can promote a more restful and rejuvenating night's sleep. 8. Promotion of General Health: Finally, the Super Metabolism Diet promotes general health and well-being through the adoption of eating habits and a healthy lifestyle. It promotes optimal nutrition, regular movement and stress management, helping to keep your body and mind healthy in the long term. In summary, the Super Metabolism Diet offers a number of tangible benefits for those looking to improve their metabolic health, lose weight in a healthy and sustainable way, and promote overall well-being.

UNDERSTANDING METABOLISM

Metabolism is one of the most fundamental processes in our body, responsible for converting the food we eat into energy that can be used to carry out our daily activities. This complex biochemical system involves a series of chemical reactions that occur within our cells, and which influence how our body uses and conserves energy. There are two main components of metabolism:
1.Catabolism: This process involves the breaking down of complex food molecules into simpler molecules, releasing energy in the process. For example, during digestion, proteins are broken down into amino acids, carbohydrates into sugars, and fats into fatty acids and glycerol.

2. Anabolism: This process involves the synthesis of complex molecules from simpler molecules, requiring energy. For example, during tissue growth and repair, cells use nutrient molecules to create new proteins, carbohydrates, and fats. Basal metabolic rate represents the amount of energy needed to maintain the body's vital functions in a resting state, such as breathing, blood circulation and body temperature. This constant energy expenditure makes up the majority of calories burned throughout the day. However, metabolism is not a static process and can vary from person to person based on a number of factors, including: Age: Metabolism tends to slow down with age, partly due to loss of muscle mass and other physiological changes. Body Composition: Muscle burns more calories than fat, so people with greater muscle mass tend to have faster metabolisms.

Genetics: Genetic predispositions can affect metabolism and the body's ability to burn calories. **Physical Activity Level:** Regular exercise can increase your metabolism and improve your body's efficiency in using energy. **Diet:** Some foods and nutrients can affect your metabolism, for example proteins require more energy to digest than carbohydrates and fats. Understanding your metabolism is critical to adopting effective weight management strategies and promoting overall health. In the next sections, we will explore how the Supermetabolism Diet can optimize the functioning of our metabolism, allowing us to achieve our health and fitness goals in a healthy and sustainable way.

THE RULES OF THE SUPER METABOLISM DIET: WHAT TO DO AND WHAT NOT TO DO

The Supermetabolism diet is a food program that involves speeding up your metabolism and burning fat through a specific food plan and exercise program.

Here are the main rules of the diet:

What to do:

Eat 5 meals a day: The diet involves dividing your daily caloric intake into 5 small meals, to keep your metabolism active and reduce hunger. Consume protein with every meal: Protein is essential for building and maintaining muscle mass, which in turn helps you burn more calories.

Choose whole foods: Give priority to fruit, vegetables, whole grains and legumes, which are rich in nutrients and fibre.

Limit saturated fats and trans fats: These fats are found primarily in red meat, full-fat dairy products and processed foods. Avoid added sugars: Added sugars are found in many processed foods, sugary drinks and sweets. Drink plenty of water: Drinking water helps you stay hydrated and feel full. Exercise regularly: Exercise is important for burning calories and increasing muscle mass. The diet suggests doing at least 30 minutes of moderate physical activity most days of the week.

What not to do:

Skipping meals: Skipping meals can slow your metabolism and lead to increased hunger and binge eating. Eating Processed Foods: Processed foods are often high in calories, saturated fat, sodium and added sugars and low in nutrients. Drinking alcohol: Alcohol is caloric and can dehydrate you.

Not getting enough sleep: Lack of sleep can slow your metabolism and increase your appetite. It is important to note that the Supermetabolism diet is not suitable for everyone. Before starting any new eating plan, it is important to consult a doctor or dietitian to ensure it is safe and effective for your individual needs. Furthermore, it is important to remember that weight loss should be a gradual and sustainable process. The Supermetabolism diet promises rapid weight loss, but it's important to be realistic and focus on long-term, healthy lifestyle changes.

THE SCIENCE BEHIND ENHANCED METABOLISM

Metabolism is one of our body's most complex and crucial processes, directly influencing our ability to burn calories, maintain a healthy weight, and promote overall health. The science behind enhanced metabolism is based on a series of physiological and biochemical principles that guide how our bodies process and use energy from the food we eat. Here are some key concepts underlying the science of enhanced metabolism: 1. Thermogenesis: This term refers to the production of heat in the body as a result of the digestion and metabolism of foods. Some foods, such as proteins, require more energy to digest and metabolize than carbohydrates and fats, thus contributing to a temporary increase in metabolism.

2. Thermal Effect of Food (TEF): TEF represents the amount of energy needed to digest, absorb and metabolize the nutrients present in the food we eat. Proteins have the highest TEF, followed by carbohydrates and fats. Incorporating an adequate amount of protein into your diet can therefore increase your metabolism through TEF. **3. Basal Metabolism:** This represents the amount of energy needed to support the body's vital functions in a resting state. Factors such as muscle mass, age and gender influence a person's basal metabolic rate. Increasing muscle mass and maintaining an active lifestyle can contribute to a higher basal metabolic rate. **4. Physical Activity:** Regular exercise not only burns calories during the activity itself, but can also increase your resting metabolism. Weight training, for example, can increase muscle mass and speed up your metabolism in the long term.

5. Hormone Regulation: Hormones such as insulin, cortisol, glucagon and catecholamines play a fundamental role in regulating metabolism, hunger and satiety. An optimal hormonal balance can promote a healthy and efficient metabolism. The Supermetabolism Diet builds on this scientific foundation to design a nutritional approach that stimulates metabolism, promotes weight loss and promotes overall health. By incorporating high-protein foods, balanced meal planning, regular exercise and stress management, we can optimize the functioning of our metabolism and achieve our wellness goals. In the following sections, we will explore practical strategies for implementing these principles into everyday life, transforming our metabolism and improving our overall health.

ASSESS YOUR CURRENT METABOLIC HEALTH

Before making any significant diet or lifestyle changes, it's important to evaluate your current metabolic health to better understand where you stand and which areas may require intervention. Here are some ways to assess your current metabolic health: 1. Blood Tests: Blood tests can provide valuable information about your metabolic health. Some common tests include fasting blood glucose to assess glucose control, lipid profile to measure cholesterol and triglyceride levels, and glycated hemoglobin (A1C) to assess long-term glucose control . 2. Blood Pressure Measurement: Elevated blood pressure is a risk factor for many chronic diseases, including heart disease and diabetes.

Measuring your blood pressure regularly can help you monitor your overall metabolic health. 3. Measuring Waist Circumference and BMI: Waist circumference and BMI (Body Mass Index) are common indicators of obesity and overweight, which can negatively affect metabolic health. Measuring your waist circumference and calculating your BMI can provide a general estimate of your metabolic health. 4. Lifestyle Assessment: Carefully examine your current lifestyle, including your eating patterns, physical activity levels, sleeping habits and stress levels. Identify any areas where you could make improvements to optimize your metabolic health. 5. Medical Consultation: If you have concerns about your metabolic health or are considering a significant change in your diet or lifestyle, it is advisable to consult your doctor or health professional.

They can help you assess your individual risks, provide personalized advice, and guide you in planning a path to better metabolic health. Once you have assessed your current metabolic health, you will be able to identify the aspects that need attention and develop a targeted action plan to improve your overall health and optimize your metabolism. In the next sections, we'll explore practical strategies and tips for implementing positive changes in your diet and lifestyle to achieve your long-term health and wellness goals.

SUPER FOODS TOSTIMULATE METABOLISM

A key component of the Super Metabolism Diet is the incorporation of superfoods that help speed up your metabolism and help you achieve your health and fitness goals. These foods are rich in essential nutrients, antioxidants, and bioactive substances that can support your metabolism and improve your overall health. Here are some superfoods to include in your diet: 1. Lean protein: Lean proteins, such as chicken, turkey, fish, eggs and low-fat dairy products, require more energy to digest and metabolize than carbohydrates and fats. Consuming an adequate amount of protein can help maintain muscle mass, speed up your metabolism and promote feelings of satiety.

2. Dark, leafy greens: Greens like spinach, kale, chard, and arugula are rich in fiber, vitamins, minerals, and antioxidants that support metabolic and overall health. Dark leafy greens are also relatively low in calories, making them a great choice for maintaining a healthy body weight. 3. Berries: Strawberries, blueberries, raspberries and other berries are rich in antioxidants, including polyphenols and anthocyanins, which can help fight inflammation and support metabolic health. Plus, they're relatively low in sugar and calories, making them a healthy and nutritious snack. 4. Chili Peppers and Spices: Chili peppers and other spices such as black pepper, ginger, turmeric, and cinnamon contain bioactive compounds that can temporarily boost your metabolism and aid in fat burning. Add a sprinkle of spices to your meals to give your metabolism a boost.

5. Legumes: Legumes such as beans, lentils and chickpeas are rich in fibre, protein and complex carbohydrates which promote satiety and regulate blood sugar levels. Consuming legumes regularly can help keep your energy level stable and support your metabolism. 6. Green Tea: Green tea is rich in catechins, antioxidants that can help boost metabolism and promote fat burning. Replace sugary drinks with a cup of green tea to enjoy its metabolic benefits. Including a variety of these superfoods in your daily diet can provide your body with the nutrients it needs to support a healthy metabolism and optimize your overall health. Try to balance your meals and snacks with a combination of proteins, complex carbohydrates, healthy fats and a variety of fruits and vegetables to maximize the benefits to your metabolism and overall well-being.

MEAL PLANNING STRATEGIES FOR A SUPER METABOLISM

Meal planning is a key element of the Super Metabolism Diet, allowing you to provide your body with the nutrients it needs to support a healthy metabolism and optimize your overall health. Here are some practical strategies for planning balanced meals that promote a super metabolism: 1. Include protein in every meal: Protein is essential for supporting muscle mass and speeding up the metabolism. Be sure to include lean protein sources such as chicken, fish, tofu, legumes and low-fat dairy products in every meal. 2. Prioritize complex carbohydrates: Choose complex carbohydrates such as quinoa, brown rice, sweet potatoes and whole grains instead of refined carbohydrates.

3. Include healthy fats: Healthy fats, like those found in avocados, nuts, seeds, olive oil, and fatty fish, are essential for metabolic health and overall well-being. Add a source of healthy fats to each meal to promote satiety and support vital body functions. 4. Eat nutritious snacks: Nutritious snacks can help keep your metabolism active and prevent excessive hunger between meals. Opt for snacks rich in protein and fiber, such as Greek yogurt with fresh fruit, raw vegetables with hummus or a handful of nuts and seeds. 5. Balance your portions: Pay attention to portion sizes to avoid calorie excess. Use smaller plates, measure portions and listen to your body's satiety signals to avoid overeating. 6. Plan ahead: Spend time planning meals and preparing foods ahead of time.

Create a weekly menu, shop for necessary ingredients, and batch prepare meals for the week. This will help you reduce stress and make healthier eating decisions throughout the week. 7. Drink plenty of water: Keeping your body hydrated is essential to supporting a healthy metabolism. Drink plenty of water during the day and limit the consumption of sugary and caloric drinks. 8. Flexibility and variety: Maintain flexibility in your diet and experiment with a variety of nutritious foods. Don't be afraid to try new recipes and healthy foods that you like. By following these meal planning strategies, you can create a balanced, sustainable diet that supports a super metabolism and promotes your overall health in the long term. Remember that balance and consistency are key to achieving lasting results and maintaining optimal well-being.

INTEGRATING PHYSICAL EXERCISE INTO YOUR LIFESTYLE LINKED TO SUPER METABOLISM

Integrating exercise into your supermetabolism lifestyle is essential to optimizing your metabolism, improving your fitness, and promoting overall well-being. Here are some ways to incorporate physical activity into your daily routine: 1. Choose activities you enjoy: Find physical activities that you enjoy and are passionate about. You might opt for outdoor walking, running, swimming, yoga, weightlifting, dancing or team sports. By choosing activities that you enjoy, you will be more likely to engage in them regularly. 2. Make exercise a priority: Schedule exercise as an integral part of your day. Find a time that works best for you, whether it's early in the morning, during your lunch break, or in the evening.

Mark workouts in your calendar and treat them as non-negotiable appointments. 3. Be consistent: Consistency is key to achieving long-lasting results. Try to exercise at least five days a week, even if it's just short training sessions. Even small increases in physical activity can make a difference in the long term. 4. Vary your routine: Alternate between different forms of exercise to prevent boredom from setting in and prevent overuse injuries. Keep your workout routine varied and interesting by including a combination of cardiovascular, resistance, flexibility and balance exercises. 5. Move more during the day: Try to be more active throughout the day, even outside of your scheduled workout sessions. Park further away, take the stairs instead of the elevator, take active breaks during work and try to move as much as possible.

6. Find a workout partner: Finding a friend, family member or colleague to workout with can be motivating and fun. Exercising with a partner can help you stay accountable and keep your motivation high. **7. Listen to your body:** Respect your body's signals and don't push yourself beyond your limits. If you feel pain or discomfort during exercise, stop and consult a health professional. **8. Celebrate your successes:** Recognize your progress and celebrate your successes, even small ones. Keep a training journal to track your improvements over time and use it as a source of motivation. By integrating exercise into your daily life, you can maximize the benefits of supermetabolism and achieve your health and fitness goals effectively and sustainably.

STRESS MANAGEMENT TECHNIQUES TO OPTIMIZE METABOLISM

Managing stress is crucial to optimizing your metabolism and improving overall well-being. Chronic stress can negatively affect metabolism, increasing cortisol levels and interfering with hormone regulation. Here are some stress management techniques that can help you support a super metabolism: 1. Meditation and Mindfulness: Meditation and mindfulness are practices that can help you reduce stress, calm the mind and promote relaxation. Dedicate a few minutes a day to meditation, focusing on your breathing and the sensations present in the present moment. 2. Physical Exercise: Regular physical activity is a powerful antidote to stress. Find a physical activity that you enjoy and that allows you to release accumulated tension.

3. Yoga: Yoga combines physical movement, mindful breathing and meditation, offering a complete form of stress management. Yoga practices can help you relax your body and mind, improve flexibility, and reduce anxiety. 4. Deep Breathing: Deep breathing can activate the parasympathetic nervous system, inducing a relaxation response in the body. Dedicate a few minutes a day to deep breathing practices, slowly inhaling and exhaling through your nose. 5. Recreational Activities: Dedicate time to activities that bring you joy and allow you to disconnect from your daily routine. Cultivate hobbies like reading, painting, music or gardening to reduce stress and renew your spirit. 6. Time outdoors: Spending time outdoors, surrounded by nature, can have calming effects on the mind and body. Take nature walks, practice yoga outdoors, or spend some time

time in the garden to regenerate and reduce stress. 7. Self-Care: Take care of your body and mind through self-care practices. Take relaxing baths with essential oils, listen to soothing music, read a book you love or treat yourself to a massage to reduce stress and rejuvenate. 8. Limit Stimuli: Reduce exposure to sources of stress, such as negative news, conflict situations or excessive use of electronic devices. Set clear limits on time spent on social media and news, and create quiet spaces in your day. By integrating these stress management techniques into your daily life, you can support a healthy metabolism and promote your overall well-being. Remember that finding the strategies that work best for you requires experimentation and patience.

SLEEP AND ITS IMPACT ON METABOLIC HEALTH

Sleep plays a critical role in metabolic health and maintaining a healthy body weight. Here's how sleep affects metabolic health: 1. Leptin is a hormone that suppresses appetite, while ghrelin stimulates appetite. Sleep deprivation can lead to decreased leptin and increased ghrelin, leading to increased appetite and a greater likelihood of overeating. 2. Blood Sugar Control: Sleep affects insulin sensitivity and blood sugar regulation. Sleep deprivation can lead to reduced insulin sensitivity, increasing the risk of developing insulin resistance and type 2 diabetes. 3. Lipid Metabolism: Sleep also affects the metabolism of lipids in the body. Sleep deprivation can lead to increased levels of lipids in the blood, such as cholesterol and triglycerides,

increasing the risk of cardiovascular disease.
4. Inflammation: Sleep affects the body's inflammatory response. Sleep deprivation can lead to increased inflammation in the body, which is associated with a number of metabolic disorders and chronic conditions.
5. Weight Control: Sleep affects body weight control. Sleep deprivation can lead to an increased tendency to accumulate body fat, particularly visceral fat, which is associated with an increased risk of obesity and metabolic disease. To improve metabolic health and promote a healthy body weight, it's important to prioritize sleep and adopt good sleep habits, including: Aim for Consistency: Try to go to bed and wake up at the same time every day, including holidays and weekends. weekend. Create a Relaxing Bedtime Routine: Create a relaxing bedtime routine, like reading a book, doing yoga, or taking a warm bath.

Limit Stimuli Before Bed: Reduce exposure to electronic devices such as smartphones, computers and television before bed, as the blue light emitted by these devices can interfere with sleep. Create a Comfortable Sleep Environment: Make sure your sleep environment is comfortable and relaxing, with a good mattress, clean sheets and a cool temperature. Limit Caffeine and Alcohol Intake: Avoid consuming caffeine and alcohol in the hours before sleep, as they can interfere with the quality of your sleep. Stay Active During the Day: Get regular physical activity during the day, but avoid exercising too close to bedtime, as it can interfere with sleep. Prioritizing sleep and adopting healthy sleep habits is essential to optimizing metabolic health, supporting a healthy body weight, and promoting overall well-being.

MONITOR YOUR PROGRESS AND ADAPT YOUR APPROACH

Tracking your progress is critical to evaluating the effectiveness of your supermetabolism approach and making any necessary adjustments. Here are some ways to monitor your progress and adapt your approach: 1.Keep a Food Diary: Record what you eat and drink each day, including main meals, snacks, portions and calories. Keeping a food diary will help you identify any problematic eating patterns and be mindful of your food choices. 2. Measure Your Physical Performance: If you're following an exercise program, record your physical performance, such as time, distance, or amount of weight lifted. Tracking your performance will help you evaluate your progress and adjust the intensity and duration of your training as needed.

3. Measure Physical Changes: Use tools like a scale, tape measure, or a measurement app to track changes in body weight, waist circumference, body measurements, and body fat percentages. Keep in mind that body weight alone may not fully reflect your progress, so it's important to consider other measurements as well. 4. Assess Your Energy Levels and Wellbeing: Pay attention to your energy levels, mood and overall well-being. If you feel fatigued, stressed, or lacking energy, you may need to review your diet, physical activity level, or sleeping habits. 5. Compare to Your Goals: Periodically, compare your progress to the goals you initially set. Consider whether you are progressing toward your goals or whether you need to make changes to your plan to achieve them more effectively.

6. Seek External Feedback: Speak to a health professional, such as a nutritionist, personal trainer, or doctor, to get objective feedback and evaluation of your progress. They can offer advice and suggestions based on your individual situation. 7. Be Flexible and Adaptable: Remember that the path to achieving your supermetabolism goals may require adaptations and adjustments along the way. Be flexible in your approach and open to trying new strategies or making changes to your plan based on your needs and results. Monitoring your progress regularly and adapting your approach to suit your needs will help you maximize the benefits of Super Metabolism and achieve your long-term health and wellness goals.

OVERCOMING COMMON CHALLENGES AND PITFALLS

Overcoming common challenges and pitfalls is an integral part of the path to supermetabolism and overall well-being. Here are some common challenges and strategies for dealing with them successfully: 1. Food Temptations: Food temptations can be difficult to resist, especially when you are exposed to indulgent foods or social situations involving food. To meet this challenge, plan ahead and prepare healthy, nutritious snacks to take with you when you're away from home. Also keep portions under control and try stress management techniques like meditation or deep breathing to reduce the urge to emotionally eat. 2. Weight Loss Stalls: It's normal to experience periods of weight loss stalls on your journey to supermetabolism. Instead of getting discouraged, focus your attention on non-weight related progress, such as improvements in physical performance or body measurements. Also rethink your diet and exercise regime to identify any areas where you can make improvements. 3. Lack of Motivation: Lack of motivation can hinder your commitment to supermetabolism. To keep motivated, set realistic, meaningful goals that inspire you. Also seek support from friends, family, or an online community who share your goals and can offer you support and encouragement. 4. Stress and Busy Lifestyle: Stress and a busy lifestyle can make it difficult to dedicate time to exercise and preparing healthy meals. Organize your time effectively and identify priorities in your life. Find ways to integrate physical activity into your daily routine, such as taking a walk during your lunch break or doing exercises at home. Also, plan meals in advance and prepare nutritious foods that you can eat on the go.

5. Frustration and Impatience: Achieving your supermetabolism goals takes time and effort. Avoid frustration and impatience by focusing on small progress and daily successes. Also celebrate your successes, even the smallest ones, and remember that every step forward brings you closer to your goals.

6. Occasional Relapses: Occasional relapses are part of the journey and should not discourage you. Accept that mistakes happen and don't let an isolated relapse undermine your overall progress. Start where you left off and commit to making healthier choices in the future. Tackling these challenges with determination, flexibility, and patience will help you overcome obstacles and progress toward your goal of supermetabolism and overall well-being. Be kind to yourself and be proud of your efforts to adopt a healthier lifestyle.

FREQUENTLY ASKED QUESTIONS AND TROUBLESHOOTING

Here are some frequently asked questions and troubleshooting questions related to the Super Metabolism Diet: 1. Why am I not losing weight despite following the Super Metabolism Diet? There could be several reasons behind this situation. You may not be in a calorie deficit, you may be eating too many calories, you may not be getting enough exercise, you may not be consistent in following your diet, or you may have health problems that affect your metabolism. Be sure to review your diet, check your portions and overall calorie intake, and evaluate your physical activity. If you have any concerns about your health, consult a medical professional. 2. How can I speed up my metabolism? You can speed up your metabolism through regular exercise, especially weight training which helps build and maintain muscle mass.

Make sure you get adequate rest and sleep, and consider incorporating metabolism-boosting foods into your diet, such as lean proteins, high-fiber foods, and spices like chili peppers. 3. What are some foods I can eat during the Super Metabolism Diet? During the Super Metabolism Diet, you can consume a variety of healthy foods, including lean proteins like chicken, fish, and tofu, complex carbohydrates like quinoa, brown rice, and sweet potatoes, healthy fats like avocado, nuts, and seeds, and a wide range of fruits and vegetables. 4. How much exercise should I do during the Super Metabolism Diet? The ideal is to do at least 150 minutes of moderate physical activity or 75 minutes of vigorous physical activity each week, along with muscular resistance exercises at least twice a week. However, your level of physical activity depends on your individual needs, health and fitness goals.

5. Can I do the supermetabolism diet if I have health problems? Before starting any diet or exercise program, it is advisable to consult a medical professional, especially if you have pre-existing health problems or are under medical treatment. A doctor can evaluate your situation and provide you with appropriate advice based on your individual needs. Addressing these frequently asked questions will help you better understand the Super Metabolism Diet and overcome any obstacles you may encounter along the way. If you have further questions or concerns, please do not hesitate to consult a health professional.

CONCLUSION EMBRACE YOUR JOURNEY INTO SUPER METABOLISM

As you conclude your supermetabolism journey, it's important to reflect on your experiences, challenges faced, and successes along the way. Embracing your supermetabolism journey means recognizing the value of your commitment to a healthier, more conscious life. During this journey, you have learned the importance of a balanced diet, rich in nutritious foods that support metabolism and overall well-being. You've explored new strategies for incorporating exercise into your daily routine, improving your fitness and vitality. Have you faced common challenges such as food temptations, stress and lack of motivation, and you have learned to overcome them with determination, flexibility and patience. You've experienced the benefits of quality sleep and stress management practices, recognizing the critical role they play in metabolic health. Now, looking back on your supermetabolism journey, you can feel proud of the progress you've made and the positive habits you've acquired along the way. Remember that your journey to health and wellness is an ongoing process, and that it's important to maintain focus and commitment for the long term. Continue to cultivate healthy lifestyle habits, explore new opportunities to improve your health, and celebrate successes, even the small ones.

Be kind to yourself during times of challenge and remember that every step forward brings you closer to your goal of a life full of vitality and well-being. May your journey into supermetabolism continue to inspire and guide you towards a life full of energy, health and happiness. And always remember to listen to your body, follow your heart, and enjoy every moment of your journey to a better version of yourself.

RECIPES APPETIZERS

QUINOA AND GRILLED VEGETABLES SALAD

Preparation time: 15 minutes

3. Cooking times: 20 minutes

4. Doses for 4 people

5. Ingredients

Quinoa: 200g

Mixed vegetables (courgettes, peppers, aubergines): 500g

Olive oil: 30g

Lemon juice: 20g

Salt and pepper to taste 6.

Preparation:

Cook the quinoa according to the package instructions. Cut the vegetables into slices and grill them on a hot griddle until tender. In a large bowl, mix the cooked quinoa with the grilled vegetables. Season with olive oil, lemon juice, salt and pepper to taste .

WHOLE WHOLE BRUSCHETTAS WITH FRESH TOMATOES AND BASIL

Preparation time: 10 minutes

Cooking times: 5 minutes

4. Doses for 4 people

5. Ingredients

Wholemeal bread: 4

slices of 50g each

Fresh tomatoes: 400g

Fresh basil: 30g

Garlic: 1 clove

Extra virgin olive oil: 30g

Salt to taste

Preparation:

Lightly toast the slices of wholemeal bread. Cut the tomatoes into cubes and chop the basil and garlic. Mix the tomatoes, basil, garlic and olive oil in a bowl. Spread the dressing over the toasted bread slices.

CHICKPEA HUMMUS WITH VEGETABLE STICKS

Preparation time: 15 minutes

Cooking times: 0 minutes

Doses for 4 people

Ingredients

Cooked chickpeas: 400g

Tahini (sesame cream): 60g

Lemon juice: 30g

Garlic: 1 clove

Extra virgin olive oil: 30g

Salt to taste

Vegetable sticks (carrots, celery, peppers): 400g

Preparation:

In a blender, combine the cooked chickpeas, tahini, lemon juice, minced garlic, olive oil and salt. Blend until you obtain a smooth and homogeneous consistency. If necessary, add a little water to reach the desired consistency. Serve the hummus with the vegetable sticks as an accompaniment.

GRILLED AUBERGINES WITH SAUCE FRESH TOMATO

Preparation time: 15 minutes

Cooking times: 15 minutes

Doses for 4 people

Ingredients

Aubergines: 600g

Fresh tomatoes: 500g

Garlic: 2 cloves

Fresh basil: 30g

Extra virgin olive oil: 40g

Salt and Pepper To Taste

Preparation:

Cut the aubergines into slices and grill them on both sides until soft and lightly browned. Cut the tomatoes into cubes and chop the garlic and basil. In a pan, heat the olive oil and fry the garlic. Add the chopped tomatoes and cook for a few minutes until the tomatoes fall apart slightly. Add the chopped basil, salt and pepper. Serve the grilled aubergines with the fresh tomato sauce on top. Be sure to customize the quantities and instructions to your preferences and dietary needs.

COURGETTE CARPACCIO WITH PARMESAN FLAKES AND BALSAMIC VINEGAR

Preparation time: 15 minutes

Cooking times: 0 minutes

Doses for 4 people, Ingredients

Courgettes: 400g Parmesan Grana: 100g

Balsamic vinegar: 30g

Extra virgin olive oil: 30g

Salt and Pepper To Taste

Preparation:

Cut the courgettes into thin slices using a mandolin or potato peeler. Arrange the courgette slices on a serving plate. Season the courgettes with olive oil, salt and pepper. Spread the parmesan flakes over the courgettes. Spray balsamic vinegar over the carpaccio just before serving.

BAKED SWEET POTATOES WITH GREEK YOGURT SAUCE AND AROMATIC HERBS

Preparation time: 15 minutes

Cooking times: 30/40 minutes

Doses for 4 people

Ingredients

Sweet potatoes: 800g

Greek yogurt: 200g

Herbs

mixed (rosemary,

thyme, parsley): 30g

Salt and Pepper To Taste

Preparation:

Preheat the oven to 200°C. Wash and cut the sweet potatoes into wedges. Place the sweet potatoes on a baking tray and drizzle with olive oil, salt, pepper and chopped herbs. Bake in the preheated oven for 30/40 minutes or until the potatoes are soft and lightly browned. Mix the Greek yogurt with the chopped aromatic herbs and a pinch of salt. Serve the sweet potatoes hot with the Greek yogurt sauce. Be sure to adjust the quantities and instructions based on your preferences and dietary needs.

AVOCADOS STUFFED
WITH TUNA AND LEMON

Preparation time: 10 minutes

Cooking times: 0 minutes

Doses for 4 people

Ingredients

Avocado: 2 large

Canned tuna: 200g

Lemon: 1, juice

and grated zest

Salt and Pepper To Taste

Preparation:

Cut the avocados in half and remove the pit. In a bowl, mix the drained tuna with the lemon juice and grated zest. Season with salt and pepper to taste. Fill the cavities of the avocados with the tuna mixture. Serve immediately as an appetizer or snack.

CHERRY TOMATOES STUFFED WITH GOAT'S CHEESE AND PARSLEY

Preparation time: 15 minutes

Cooking times: 0 minutes

Doses for 4 people

Ingredients

Cherry tomatoes: 200g

Goat cheese: 100g

Fresh parsley: 20g,

finely chopped

Salt and Pepper To Taste

Preparation:

Cut off the tops of the cherry tomatoes and hollow them out gently with a teaspoon. In a bowl, mash the goat cheese with the chopped parsley. Season with salt and pepper to taste. Fill the cherry tomatoes with the goat cheese mixture. Serve as an appetizer or as a fresh and tasty side dish.

BUFFALO MOZZARELLA WITH TOMATOES AND FRESH BASIL

Preparation time: 10 minutes

Cooking times: 0 minutes

Doses for 4 people

Ingredients

Buffalo mozzarella: 250g

Cherry tomatoes: 200g

Fresh basil: 20g

Extra virgin olive oil: 30ml

Salt and Pepper To Taste

Preparation:

Cut the buffalo mozzarella into thick slices.
Cut the cherry tomatoes in half. Arrange the
mozzarella slices on a serving plate. Spread
the cherry tomatoes over the mozzarella
slices. Sprinkle with fresh basil leaves.
Season with extra virgin olive oil, salt and
pepper to taste. Serve as a fresh and tasty
appetizer.

RAW VEGETABLES WITH YOGURT SAUCE AND FRESH HERBS

Preparation time: 15 minutes

Cooking times: 0 minutes

Doses for 4 people

Ingredients

Raw mixed vegetables (carrots, celery, peppers, cucumbers): 400g

Greek yogurt: 200g

Mixed fresh herbs (parsley, mint, chives): 30g

Lemon juice: 20ml

Salt and pepper

Preparation:

Wash and cut raw vegetables into sticks or slices. In a bowl, mix the Greek yogurt with the chopped fresh herbs and lemon juice. Season with salt and pepper according to your taste. Serve the raw vegetables with the yogurt sauce as a condiment. Be sure to adjust the quantities and instructions based on your preferences and dietary needs.

QUINOA FRITTERS WITH MIXED VEGETABLES

Preparation time: 20 minutes

Cooking times: 15 minutes

Doses for 4 people

Ingredients

Cooked quinoa: 300g

Mixed vegetables (courgettes, carrots, peppers): 200g

Eggs: 2

Chickpea flour: 50g

Fresh parsley: 20g, chopped

Salt and Pepper To Taste

Olive oil for cooking

Preparation:

In a bowl, mix the cooked quinoa with the diced mixed vegetables, eggs, chickpea flour and chopped parsley. Season with salt and pepper to taste. Form pancakes with the mixture obtained. Heat the olive oil in a non-stick pan and cook the pancakes until golden on both sides. Serve hot as a side dish or main course.

QUINOA SALAD WITH GRILLED CHICKEN

Preparation time: 15 minutes

Cooking times: 20 minutes

Doses for 4 people

Ingredients

Quinoa: 200g

Chicken breast: 400g

Mixed vegetables (tomatoes, cucumbers, peppers): 300g

Black olives: 50g

Lemon juice: 30ml

Extra virgin olive oil: 50ml

Salt and Pepper To Taste

Preparation:

Cook the quinoa according to the package instructions and let it cool. Cut the chicken breast into slices and grill until fully cooked. Cut the vegetables into cubes and the olives into slices. In a large bowl, mix the cooked quinoa, grilled chicken, mixed greens and olives. Season with lemon juice, olive oil, salt and pepper. Mix well and serve as a main dish or side dish.

WHOLE BREAD CANAPÉS WITH AVOCADO PESTO

Preparation time: 15 minutes

Cooking times: 0 minutes

Doses for 4 people

Ingredients

Sliced wholemeal bread: 8 slices

Ripe avocado: 2

Lemon juice: 20ml

Garlic: 1 clove

Fresh basil: 30g

Salt and Pepper To Taste

Preparation:

Lightly toast the slices of wholemeal bread. In a bowl, mash the avocados with the lemon juice, minced garlic and fresh basil. Season with salt and pepper to taste. Spread the avocado pesto on the toasted bread slices. Serve as an appetizer or snack.

LENTIL MEATBALLS WITH YOGURT AND MINT SAUCE

Preparation time: 20 minutes

Cooking times: 20 minutes

Doses for 4 people

Ingredients

Dried lentils: 200g

Red onion: 1 small

Garlic: 2 cloves

Fresh parsley: 30g, chopped

Egg: 1

Chickpea flour: 50g

Greek yogurt: 200g

Fresh mint: 20g, chopped

Salt and Pepper To Taste

Preparation:

Boil the lentils in boiling water until soft, then drain and mash with a fork. Finely chop the onion and garlic and add them to the lentils together with the parsley, egg and chickpea flour. Mix the mixture well and form meatballs. Cook the meatballs in a non-stick pan until golden on both sides. Mix the Greek yogurt with the chopped mint and season with salt and pepper. Serve the meatballs with the yogurt and mint sauce as an accompaniment.

MUSHROOM CARPACCIO WITHEXTRA VIRGIN OLIVE OIL AND LEMON

Preparation time: 10 minutes

Cooking times: 0 minutes

Doses for 4 people

Ingredients

Fresh mushrooms

(porcini, mushrooms,

or other mushrooms

of your choice): 200g

Extra virgin olive oil: 30ml

Lemon: 1, juice

Salt and Pepper To Taste

Parmesan flakes (optional)

Preparation:

Clean the mushrooms carefully and slice them finely. Arrange the mushroom slices on a serving plate. Season with extra virgin olive oil and lemon juice. Season with salt and pepper to taste. If necessary, add some flakes of parmesan to decorate. Serve as a fresh and light appetizer.

CROSTINI WITH CREAM OF WITHEBEANS AND ROSEMARY

Preparation time: 15 minutes

Cooking times: 10 minutes

Doses for 4 people

Ingredients

Canned white beans: 400g

Baguette bread or Tuscan bread:

1 baguette or 4 thick slices

Fresh rosemary: 10g,

finely chopped

Garlic: 2 cloves

Extra virgin olive oil: 50ml

Salt and Pepper To Taste

Preparation:

Heat the extra virgin olive oil in a pan and brown the whole garlic cloves. Add the drained white beans and heat them slightly. Remove the garlic cloves and mash the beans with a fork. Add the chopped rosemary and season with salt and pepper. Cut the bread into slices and toast it lightly. Spread the white bean cream on the bread slices. Serve the crostini hot as an appetizer or appetizer.

MIXED BEAN SALAD WITH RED ONION AND PARSLEY

Preparation time: 15 minutes

Cooking times: 0 minutes

Doses for 4 people

Ingredients

Canned mixed beans

(cannellini, borlotti, black): 400g

Red onion: 1 large

Fresh parsley: 30g, chopped

Lemon juice: 30ml

Extra virgin olive oil: 30ml

Salt and Pepper To Taste

Preparation:

Drain and rinse the mixed beans under running water. Thinly slice the red onion. In a large bowl, combine the mixed beans, red onion and chopped parsley. Season with lemon juice, extra virgin olive oil, salt and pepper. Mix all the ingredients well. Leave to rest in the refrigerator for at least 30 minutes before serving. Serve as a fresh and tasty side dish.

COURGETTE ROLL WITH RICOTTA AND DRIED TOMATOES

Preparation time: 20 minutes

Cooking times: 15 minutes

Doses for 4 people

Ingredients

Courgettes: 4 medium

Fresh ricotta: 200g

Dried tomatoes: 50g

Grated parmesan: 30g

Fresh parsley: 20g, chopped

Salt and Pepper To Taste

Extra virgin olive oil

olive for cooking

Preparation:

Cut off the ends of the courgettes and slice them lengthwise using a mandolin or potato peeler. Cook the courgette slices on a hot grill for about 23 minutes per side, until soft but still firm. In a bowl, mix the ricotta with the chopped dried tomatoes, grated Parmesan, parsley, salt and pepper. Spread a little ricotta filling on each courgette slice and roll them up. Place the rolls on a baking tray lightly greased with oil. Bake in a preheated oven at 180°C for about 10/15 minutes, until golden. Serve hot as an appetizer or main course.

PUMPKIN SOUP WITH TOASTED PUMPKIN SEEDS

Preparation time: 15 minutes

Cooking times: 30 minutes

Doses for 4 people

Ingredients

Pumpkin: 800g, peeled

and cut into cubes

Onion: 1 large, chopped

Potatoes: 2 medium, peeled

and cut into cubes

Vegetable broth: 1 litre

Fresh cream: 100ml, Butter: 2 tablespoons

Pumpkin seeds: 50g, toasted

Salt and Pepper To Taste

Preparation:

In a large pot, sauté the onion in the butter until translucent. Add the pumpkin and potatoes, and cook for about 5 minutes. Pour the vegetable broth into the pot and bring to the boil. Reduce the heat and leave to simmer for about 20/25 minutes, until the vegetables are tender. Blend the soup until it reaches a velvety consistency. Add the fresh cream and mix well. Season with salt and pepper to your taste. Serve the pumpkin soup hot, garnished with toasted pumpkin seeds.

BAKED AUBERGINE MEATBALLS WITH TOMATO SAUCE

Preparation time: 30 minutes

Cooking times: 30 minutes

Doses for 4 people

Ingredients

Aubergine: 2 medium, cut into cubes

Grated bread: 100g

Grated parmesan: 50g

Eggs: 2

Fresh parsley: 30g, chopped

Garlic: 2 cloves, minced

Tomato sauce: 500ml

Salt and Pepper To Taste

Preparation:

Preheat the oven to 180°C. Arrange the aubergine cubes on a baking tray lined with baking paper and bake in the oven for approximately 2025 minutes, until the aubergines are soft. In a large bowl, mash the cooked eggplant with a fork and add the breadcrumbs, grated Parmesan, eggs, parsley, garlic, salt and pepper. Mix the mixture well until all the ingredients are incorporated. Form meatballs with your hands and place them on a lightly greased baking tray. Cook in the preheated oven for about 25/30 minutes, until the meatballs are golden and crispy. Heat the tomato sauce in a pan and add the meatballs before serving. Serve the hot aubergine meatballs with the tomato sauce.

BLACK BEAN SALAD WITH CORN AND PEPPERS

Preparation time: 15 minutes

Cooking times: 0 minutes

Doses for 4 people

Ingredients

Canned black beans: 400g

Canned corn: 200g

Red and yellow peppers: 2,

cut into cubes

Red onion: 1 small,

finely chopped

Fresh coriander: 30g, chopped

Lime juice: 30ml

Extra virgin olive oil: 30ml

Salt and Pepper To Taste

Preparation:

In a large bowl, combine the drained and rinsed black beans, drained corn, diced peppers, and chopped red onion. Add the chopped fresh coriander. Season with lime juice, olive oil, salt and pepper. Mix gently until the ingredients are well combined. Leave to rest in the refrigerator for at least 30 minutes before serving. Serve as a fresh and colorful side dish or main course.

GRILLED VEGETABLES WITH AVOCADO AND LIME SAUCE

Preparation time: 20 minutes

Cooking times: 10 minutes

Doses for 4 people

Ingredients

Courgettes: 2 medium,

cut into long slices

Eggplant: 1 large,

cut into long slices

Red and yellow peppers:

2, cut into strips

Ripe avocado: 1 large

Lime juice: 30ml

Fresh parsley: 20g, chopped

Salt and Pepper To Taste

Preparation:

Preheat a grill or grill pan. Grill the courgette, aubergine and pepper slices until soft and lightly browned on both sides. While the vegetables are grilling, prepare the avocado salsa. In a bowl, mash the ripe avocado with a fork and mix with the lime juice and chopped fresh parsley. Season with salt and pepper to taste. Arrange the grilled vegetables on a serving platter and serve with the avocado-lime salsa. Grilled vegetables can be served hot or at room temperature as a side dish or main course.

CREAM OF CARROT WITH GINGER AND CUMIN

Preparation time: 15 minutes

Cooking times: 25 minutes

Doses for 4 people

Ingredients

Carrots: 500g, peeled

and cut into rounds

Onion: 1 large, chopped

Fresh ginger: 20g, grated

Cumin powder: 1 teaspoon

Vegetable broth: 1 litre

Fresh cream: 100ml

Extra virgin olive oil: 2 tablespoons

Salt and Pepper To Taste

Preparation:

In a large pot, heat the olive oil and sauté the onion until translucent. Add the carrots cut into slices and cook for about 5 minutes. Add grated ginger and cumin powder and mix well. Pour the vegetable broth into the pan and bring to the boil. Reduce the heat and leave to simmer for about 15/20 minutes, until the carrots are tender. Using an immersion blender, blend the soup until smooth. Add the fresh cream and mix well. Season with salt and pepper to your taste. Serve the carrot cream hot, garnished with a sprinkle of black pepper.

BRUSCHETTE WITH BEAN BEAN CREAM AND GRATED PECORINO

Preparation time: 20 minutes

Cooking times: 10 minutes

Doses for 4 people

Ingredients

Fresh or frozen broad beans: 400g

Rustic bread (baguette

or ciabatta): 4 thick slices

Grated pecorino: 50g

Extra virgin olive oil: 2 tablespoons

Garlic: 1 clove, peeled

Fresh mint: 20g, chopped

Salt and Pepper To Taste

Preparation:

Boil the broad beans in boiling water for about 5 minutes if fresh, or follow the instructions on the package if frozen. Drain them and rinse them under cold water. Peel the broad beans if fresh. In a blender, combine the boiled broad beans, garlic, fresh mint, grated pecorino, olive oil, salt and pepper. Blend until you obtain a smooth cream. Toast the bread slices in a pan or on the grill until crispy and lightly browned. Spread the broad bean cream on each slice of toasted bread. Serve the bruschetta with broad bean cream hot or at room temperature as an appetizer or appetizer.

SEAFOOD SALAD WITH TOMATOES AND PARSLEY

Preparation time: 15 minutes

Cooking times: 5 minutes

Doses for 4 people

Ingredients

Mixed seafood (mussels,

clams, shrimp):

500g, already cooked and shelled

Cherry tomatoes: 200g, cut in half

Fresh parsley: 30g, chopped

Lemon juice: 30ml

Extra virgin olive oil: 2 tablespoons

Garlic: 2 cloves, minced

Salt and Pepper To Taste

Preparation:

In a pan, heat the olive oil and fry the chopped garlic for a few minutes. Add the already cooked and shelled seafood and sauté for about 3/5 minutes, until hot. Transfer the seafood to a large bowl and let cool slightly. Add halved cherry tomatoes and chopped fresh parsley to the seafood. Season with lemon juice, salt and pepper to taste. Gently mix all the ingredients. Leave to cool completely in the refrigerator before serving. Serve the seafood salad as a fresh and tasty appetizer or main course.

CROSTINI WITH CHICKPEA CREAM AND CHILI PEPPER

Preparation time: 15 minutes

Cooking times: 10 minutes

Doses for 4 people

Ingredients

Canned chickpeas: 400g,

drained and rinsed

Rustic bread (baguette

or ciabatta): 4 thick slices

Fresh chili pepper:

1, finely chopped

Garlic: 1 clove, minced

Fresh rosemary: 1 sprig, chopped

Extra virgin olive oil: 3 tablespoons

Salt and Pepper To Taste

Preparation:

In a pan, heat 1 tablespoon of olive oil and fry the chopped garlic and chilli for a few minutes. Add the drained and rinsed chickpeas and the chopped fresh rosemary. Cook for about 57 minutes, until the chickpeas are hot and blend well with the aromas. Transfer the chickpeas into a bowl and mash them with a fork until they obtain a creamy consistency. Toast the bread slices in a pan or on the grill until crispy and lightly browned. Spread the chickpea cream on each slice of toasted bread. Season with a drizzle of olive oil, salt and pepper. Serve the crostini with hot chickpea cream as an appetizer.

BROCCOLI FLAN WITH FRESH CHEESE

Preparation time: 20 minutes

Cooking times: 30 minutes

Doses for 4 people

Ingredients

Broccoli: 500g, cleaned

and cut into florets

Eggs: 3

Fresh cheese: 200g, ricotta type

Grated parmesan: 50g

Milk: 100ml

Butter: 20g (to grease the pan)

Nutmeg: to taste, grated

Salt and Pepper To Taste

Preparation:

Cook the broccoli in boiling salted water until soft but not mushy, about 5/7 minutes. Drain the broccoli well and chop finely. In a bowl, beat the eggs with the fresh cheese, the grated parmesan and the milk. Add the chopped broccoli to the mixture and mix well. Season with a pinch of nutmeg, salt and pepper. Butter a baking tray and pour in the broccoli mixture. Level the surface with a spatula. Bake in a preheated oven at 180°C for approximately 25/30 minutes, until the flan is golden on the surface and well cooked in the centre. Once cooked, let cool slightly before serving. Serve the broccoli casserole hot as a side dish or main dish.

SWEET AND SOUR VEGETABLES WITH BALSAMIC VINEGAR

Preparation time: 15 minutes

Cooking times: 15 minutes

Doses for 4 people

Ingredients

Eggplants: 2 medium,

cut into cubes

Red and yellow peppers:

2, cut into strips

Red onion: 1 large,

sliced thinly

Balsamic vinegar: 60ml

Brown sugar: 2 tablespoons

Extra virgin olive oil: 3 tablespoons

Salt and Pepper To Taste

Preparation:

In a pan, heat the olive oil and sauté the red onion until translucent. Add the chopped aubergines and peppers and cook over medium heat for about 10 minutes, stirring occasionally. In a small bowl, mix the balsamic vinegar with the brown sugar until the sugar has completely dissolved. Pour the balsamic vinegar and sugar mixture into the pan with the vegetables and mix well. Continue to cook for another 5 minutes, until the vegetables are tender and the sauce has thickened slightly. Season with salt and pepper to your taste. Transfer the sweet and sour vegetables to a serving dish and serve hot or at room temperature as a side dish or appetizer.

QUINOA AND CHEESE CROQUETTES

Preparation time: 20 minutes

Cooking times: 25 minutes

Doses for 4 people

Ingredients

Quinoa: 200g, already cooked

Grated cheese (cheddar, parmesan, or other): 100g

Egg: 1 large

Breadcrumbs: 50g

Onion: 1 small, finely chopped

Fresh parsley: 2 spoons, finely chopped

Salt and Pepper To Taste

Extra virgin olive oil: for cooking

Preparation:

In a large bowl, combine the cooked quinoa, grated cheese, egg, breadcrumbs, chopped onion and fresh parsley. Season with salt and pepper to your taste. Mix all the ingredients well until you obtain a homogeneous mixture. Form balls with your hands and crush them lightly to create croquettes. In a nonstick pan, heat some olive oil over medium heat. Cook the quinoa and cheese croquettes for about 3/4 minutes per side, until they are golden and crispy. Once cooked, transfer them to a plate lined with absorbent paper to remove excess oil. Serve the quinoa and cheese croquettes hot as an appetizer or main course.

SPINACH SALAD WITH ALMONDS AND FETA

Preparation time: 10 minutes

Cooking times: 0 minutes

Doses for 4 people

Ingredients

Fresh spinach: 200g,

washed and dried

Almonds: 50g,

toasted and sliced

Feta: 100g, cut into cubes

Cherry tomatoes:

150g, cut in half

Lemon juice: 2 tablespoons

Extra virgin olive oil: 3 tablespoons

Salt and Pepper To Taste

Preparation:

In a large bowl, combine fresh spinach, toasted almonds, diced feta and halved cherry tomatoes. Season with lemon juice, olive oil, salt and pepper. Gently mix all the ingredients until the spinach is well seasoned. Make sure the feta and almonds are evenly distributed in the salad. Serve the spinach salad with almonds and feta as a fresh and tasty side dish or main course.

ARTICHOKE FRITTERS WITH MINT AND LEMON

Preparation time: 20 minutes

Cooking times: 10 minutes

Doses for 4 people

Ingredients

Artichokes: 4, cleaned and

sliced thinly

Flour: 100g Eggs: 2

Fresh mint: 2

spoons, finely chopped

Lemon peel

grated: from 1 lemon

Salt and Pepper To Taste

Extra olive oil

virgin: for cooking

Preparation:

In a bowl, mix the flour, beaten eggs, chopped fresh mint and grated lemon zest. Add salt and pepper to your taste and mix until you get a smooth batter. Add the artichoke slices to the batter and mix gently until well coated. In a nonstick pan, heat some olive oil over medium heat. Using a spoon, scoop out some of the batter with a piece of artichoke and pour it into the hot pan. Cook the artichoke fritters for about 3/4 minutes per side, until they are golden and crispy. Once cooked, transfer them to a plate lined with absorbent paper to remove excess oil. Serve the artichoke fritters hot as an appetizer or side dish.

CAPRESE WITH BUFFALO MOZZARELLA AND OX HEART TOMATOES

Preparation time: 10 minutes

Cooking times: 0 minutes

Doses for 4 people

Ingredients

Buffalo mozzarella:

250g, cut into slices

Ox heart tomatoes:

4 large, cut into slices

Fresh basil: a few leaves

Extra virgin olive oil: 3 tablespoons

Balsamic vinegar: 2 tablespoons

Salt and Pepper To Taste

Preparation:

1. Arrange the buffalo mozzarella slices and the Cuore di Bue tomatoes alternately on a serving plate, creating a fan pattern. 2. Scatter a few fresh basil leaves over the mozzarella and tomatoes. 3. Season with extra virgin olive oil, salt and freshly ground black pepper to taste. 4. If desired, add a splash of balsamic reduction for a more refined presentation. 5. Serve the Caprese immediately as an appetizer or as a fresh, light side dish.

CROSTINI WITH AUBERGINE PARMESAN

Preparation time: 20 minutes

Cooking times: 30 minutes

Doses for 4 people

Ingredients

Aubergine: 2 large,

cut into thin slices

Rustic bread (baguette or ciabatta):

8 thick slices

Peeled tomatoes: 400g, crushed

Mozzarella: 200g, cut into thin slices

Grated parmesan: 50g

Fresh basil: a few leaves

Extra virgin olive oil: 4 tablespoons

Garlic: 2 cloves, minced

Salt and Pepper To Taste

Preparation:

Preheat the oven to 180°C. Arrange the aubergine slices on a baking tray lined with baking paper, brush with a little olive oil and bake in the oven for around 15/20 minutes, until soft and lightly golden. In a pan, heat a little olive oil and fry the chopped garlic. Add the crushed peeled tomatoes and cook for about 10/15 minutes, until the sauce has thickened slightly. Toast the bread slices in the oven or on the grill until crispy. Spread a little tomato sauce on each slice of toast. Arrange a slice of roasted eggplant on top of the tomato sauce. Add a slice of mozzarella on top of the aubergines. Sprinkle with grated parmesan and decorate with fresh basil leaves. Bake the croutons for about 10 minutes, until the cheese is melted and lightly golden. Serve the crostini with aubergine parmigiana hot as an appetizer or appetizer.

AVOCADO MANGO AND PRAWNS SALAD,

Preparation time: 15 minutes

Cooking times: 0 minutes

Doses for 4 people

Ingredients

Peeled prawns :

300g, cooked and cold

Ripe avocado:

2 large, cut into cubes

Ripe mango: 1 large,

cut into cubes

Lettuce or arugula: 150g,

washed and cut into pieces

Red onion: 1 small,

sliced thinly

Fresh chili pepper: 1,

finely chopped (optional)

Lime juice: 2 tablespoons

Extra virgin olive oil: 3 tablespoons

Salt and Pepper To Taste

Preparation:

In a large bowl, combine the peeled shrimp, diced avocado, diced mango, lettuce or arugula, and sliced red onion. Add chopped fresh chili pepper, if desired, for a spicy kick. Season with lime juice, olive oil, serve.

PEAS CREAM WITH FRESH MINT

Preparation time: 15 minutes

Cooking times: 15 minutes

Doses for 4 people

Ingredients

Fresh or frozen peas: 400g

Onion: 1 medium, chopped

Vegetable broth: 500ml

Fresh mint: 10 leaves,

plus some for garnish

Cooking cream: 100ml (optional)

Salt and Pepper To Taste

Extra olive oil

virgin: 2 tbsp

Preparation:

In a saucepan, heat the olive oil and sauté the onion until translucent. Add the peas and cook for about 2 minutes. Pour the vegetable broth into the pot and bring to the boil. Reduce the heat and simmer for about 10 to 12 minutes, until the peas are tender. Add the fresh mint leaves and mix. Using an immersion blender, blend the soup until smooth and velvety. If desired, add cooking cream to obtain a creamier consistency. Season with salt and pepper to your taste. Serve the pea cream hot, garnished with fresh mint leaves.

CROSTINI WITH RICOTTA CREAM AND TAGGIASCA OLIVES

Preparation time: 10 minutes

Cooking times: 0 minutes

Doses for 4 people

Ingredients

Rustic bread (baguette

or ciabatta): 8 thick slices

Ricotta: 200g

Taggiasca olives: 50g,

pitted and chopped

Fresh parsley: 2 tablespoons,

finely chopped

Lemon peel

grated: from 1 lemon

Salt and Pepper To Taste

Extra olive oil

virgin: for the garnish

Preparation:

Toast the bread slices in the oven or on the grill until crispy. In a bowl, mix the ricotta with the chopped Taggiasca olives, the chopped fresh parsley and the grated lemon zest. Season with salt and pepper to taste and mix well. Distribute the ricotta and olive cream evenly on the toasted bread slices. Garnish each crostini with a drizzle of extra virgin olive oil. Serve the crostini with ricotta cream and olives as an appetizer or appetizer.

FENNEL ORANGES AND BLACK OLIVES SALAD

Preparation time: 15 minutes

Cooking times: 0 minutes

Doses for 4 people

Ingredients

Fennel: 2 large, cut into thin slices

Oranges: 2 large, peeled and cut into thin slices

Black olives: 100g, pitted and cut into rounds

Fresh parsley: 2 tablespoons, finely chopped

Grated lemon zest: from 1 lemon

Lemon juice: 3 tablespoons

Extra virgin olive oil: 3 tablespoons

Salt and Pepper To Taste

Preparation:

In a large bowl, combine the fennel slices, orange slices, and black olives. Add the chopped fresh parsley and the grated lemon zest. Season with lemon juice, olive oil, salt and pepper. Gently mix all ingredients until well seasoned. Make sure the ingredients are evenly distributed in the salad. Serve the fennel, orange and black olive salad as a fresh and tasty side dish or main course.

SWEET POTATO AND QUINOA CROQUETTES

Preparation time: 30 minutes

Cooking times: 25 minutes

Doses for 4 people

Ingredients

Sweet potatoes: 2 medium,

peeled and cut into cubes

Cooked quinoa: 1 cup

Onion: 1 medium, chopped

Egg: 1 large

Almond flour or breadcrumbs: 50g

Paprika: 1 tsp

Cumin: 1 tsp

Salt and Pepper To Taste

Extra olive oil virgin: for cooking

Preparation:

Boil sweet potato cubes in salted water until soft, about 10 minutes. Drain and mash the potatoes. In a large bowl, combine mashed sweet potatoes, cooked quinoa, chopped onion, beaten egg, almond flour or breadcrumbs, paprika, cumin, salt and pepper. Mix all the ingredients well until a homogeneous mixture is formed. Form balls with your hands and crush them lightly to create croquettes. In a nonstick pan, heat some olive oil over medium heat. Cook the sweet potato and quinoa croquettes for about 34 minutes per side, until golden and crispy. Once cooked, transfer them to a plate lined with absorbent paper to remove excess oil. Serve the sweet potato and quinoa croquettes hot as an appetizer.

SALAD OF TOMATOES CUCUMBERS AND BASIL

Preparation time: 10 minutes

Cooking times: 0 minutes

Doses for 4 people

Ingredients

Ripe tomatoes: 4

large, cut into slices

Cucumbers: 2 medium,

cut into thin slices

Fresh basil leaves:

1 bunch, whole

Red onion: 1 small,

thinly sliced (optional)

Extra virgin olive oil: 3 tablespoons

Red wine vinegar: 2 tablespoons

Salt and Pepper To Taste

Preparation:

In a large salad bowl, arrange the tomato and cucumber slices. Add fresh basil leaves and sliced red onion, if desired. Season with extra virgin olive oil and red wine vinegar. Add salt and pepper to your taste. Gently mix all ingredients until well seasoned. Make sure the ingredients are evenly distributed in the salad. Serve the tomato, cucumber and basil salad as a fresh and colorful side dish.

CROSTINI WITH AUBERGINE CREAM AND GREEN OLIVES

Preparation time: 20 minutes

Cooking times: 20 minutes

Doses for 4 people

Ingredients

Aubergine: 2 medium, cut into cubes

Green olives: 50g,

pitted and chopped

Garlic: 2 cloves, finely chopped

Fresh basil: a few leaves

Rustic bread (baguette

or ciabatta): 8 thick slices

Extra olive oil

virgin: 4 tbsp

Salt and Pepper To Taste

Preparation:

Preheat the oven to 180°C. Arrange the aubergine cubes on a baking tray lined with baking paper and season with a little olive oil, salt and pepper. Bake the aubergines in the preheated oven for about 20 minutes, until soft and lightly browned. In a pan, heat some olive oil and fry the minced garlic until golden. Add the chopped green olives and fresh basil leaves. Cook for another 2/3 minutes. In a blender, combine the roasted eggplant and olive-garlic mixture. Blend until you obtain a smooth and homogeneous cream. Toast the bread slices in the oven or on the grill until crispy. Spread the aubergine and olive cream on each slice of toasted bread. Serve the crostini with aubergine cream and olives as an appetizer or appetizer.

RECIPES
FIRST DISHES

MIXED VEGETABLE SOUP WITH LEGUMES

Preparation time: 15 minutes

Cooking times: 30 minutes

Doses for 4 people

Ingredients

Mixed vegetables (carrots, celery, courgettes, cabbage, potatoes): 500g, cut into cubes

Mixed legumes (chickpeas, beans, lentils): 200g, cooked

Onion: 1 medium, chopped

Garlic: 2 cloves, finely chopped

Vegetable broth: 1 litre

Peeled tomatoes: 400g, crushed

Fresh parsley: 2

spoons, finely chopped

Extra virgin olive oil: 2 tablespoons

Salt and Pepper To Taste

Preparation:

In a large saucepan, heat the olive oil and sauté the onion and garlic until golden brown. Add the diced vegetables and cook for a few minutes until they start to soften. Add the crushed peeled tomatoes and the vegetable broth. Bring the soup to the boil, then reduce the heat and leave to simmer for about 20 to 25 minutes, until the vegetables are tender. Add the cooked legumes and chopped fresh parsley. Continue to cook for another 5 minutes to allow the flavors to blend. Season with salt and pepper according to your taste. Serve the mixed vegetable soup with legumes hot, perhaps accompanied by croutons.

WHOLE WHOLE SPAGHETTI WITH FRESH TOMATO AND BASIL

Preparation time: 10 minutes

Cooking times: 15 minutes

Doses for 4 people

Ingredients

Wholemeal spaghetti: 400g

Fresh tomatoes: 6

large, cut into cubes

Garlic: 2 cloves, finely chopped

Fresh basil: 1 bunch,

leaves removed and chopped

Extra virgin olive oil: 4 tablespoons

Salt and Pepper To Taste

Preparation:

Bring a pot of salted water to a boil and cook the whole-wheat spaghetti according to package instructions until al dente. While the spaghetti is cooking, in a large skillet, heat the olive oil and sauté the minced garlic until golden brown. Add the diced fresh tomatoes and cook for about 8/10 minutes, until they begin to fall apart and form a sauce. Add half of the chopped fresh basil to the tomato sauce. Drain the spaghetti al dente and transfer them directly to the pan with the tomato and basil sauce. Sauté the spaghetti with the tomato sauce for about 1/2 minutes over medium-high heat, until they are well seasoned. Season with salt and pepper according to your taste. Serve the wholemeal spaghetti with fresh tomato and basil hot, garnished with the remaining fresh basil.

WHOLE WHOLE RISOTTO WITH PORCINI MUSHROOMS

Preparation time: 10 minutes

Cooking times: 30 minutes

Doses for 4 people

Ingredients

Brown rice: 300g

Fresh porcini mushrooms or dried: 200g, cut into slices

Vegetable broth: 1 litre

Onion: 1 medium, finely chopped

Garlic: 2 cloves, finely chopped

Dry white wine: 120ml

Grated parmesan: 50g

Butter: 2 tablespoons

Extra virgin olive oil: 2 tablespoons

Salt and Pepper To Taste

Preparation:

In a saucepan, heat the vegetable broth and keep warm over low heat. In a large skillet, heat the olive oil and butter over medium heat. Add the onion and garlic and fry until golden. Add the porcini mushrooms and cook until golden and soft. Add the brown rice to the pan and toast it lightly for a couple of minutes, stirring constantly. Pour the white wine into the pan and let it evaporate completely. Gradually add the hot vegetable broth to the rice, one ladle at a time, stirring continuously and adding more broth only when the previous one has been absorbed.

Continue cooking the risotto for about 25/30 minutes, until the rice is cooked al dente and has absorbed most of the broth. Once the risotto is cooked, remove from the heat and stir in the grated Parmesan. Season with salt and pepper according to your taste. Serve the wholemeal risotto with porcini mushrooms hot, garnished with fresh parsley if desired.

WHOLEMEWHEAT PENNE WITH ARUGULA PESTO AND WALNUTS

Preparation time: 15 minutes

Cooking times: 10 minutes

Doses for 4 people

Ingredients

Wholemeal penne: 400g

Fresh Arugula: 100g

Walnuts: 50g, toasted

Grated parmesan: 50g

Garlic: 1 clove

Extra olive oil

virgin: 4 tbsp

Salt and Pepper To Taste

Preparation:

Cook the wholemeal penne in salted water following the instructions on the package, until al dente. In the meantime, prepare the Arugula and walnut pesto. In a blender, combine the arugula, toasted walnuts, grated Parmesan, garlic and olive oil. Blend until you obtain a smooth and homogeneous consistency. Drain the whole penne, keeping a little of the cooking water. In a large bowl, season the drained penne with the Arugula and walnut pesto, adding a little of the pasta cooking water to obtain a creamy consistency. Toss the penne well with the pesto until evenly seasoned. Season with salt and pepper according to your taste. Serve the wholemeal penne with hot Arugula pesto and walnuts, garnished with some chopped walnuts and fresh Arugula leaves.

LENTIL SOUP WITH CARROTS AND CELERY

Preparation time: 10 minutes

Cooking times: 40 minutes

Doses for 4 people

Ingredients

Dried lentils: 250g,

rinse and drain

Carrots: 2 medium, diced

Celery: 2 stalks, diced

Onion: 1 medium, chopped

Garlic: 2 cloves, finely chopped

Vegetable broth: 1 litre

Peeled tomatoes: 400g, chopped

Bay leaves: 2/3 leaves

Fresh thyme: 1 teaspoon, chopped

Extra virgin olive oil: 2 tablespoons

Salt and Pepper To Taste

Preparation:

In a large saucepan, heat the olive oil and sauté the onion and garlic until golden brown. Add the diced carrots and celery and cook for a few minutes until they start to soften. Add the rinsed and drained lentils, chopped peeled tomatoes, vegetable broth, bay leaves and fresh thyme. Bring the soup to the boil, then reduce the heat and simmer for about 30 to 35 minutes, until the lentils are soft. Season with salt and pepper according to your taste. Serve the lentil soup with carrots and celery hot, perhaps accompanied by croutons.

WHOLE WHOLE PASTA SALAD WITH TOMATOES AND TUNA

Preparation time: 15 minutes

Cooking times: 10 minutes

Doses for 4 people

Ingredients

Short wholemeal pasta

(pens, fusilli, etc.): 400g

Cherry tomatoes: 250g, cut in half

Tuna in oil: 200g, drained and crumbled

Black olives: 50g, pitted and cut into rounds

Red onion: 1 small, thinly sliced

Fresh parsley: 2 tablespoons, finely chopped

Extra virgin olive oil: 4 tablespoons

Lemon juice: 2 tablespoons

Salt and Pepper To Taste

Preparation:

Cook the wholemeal pasta in salted water following the instructions on the package, until al dente. Drain the pasta and rinse it under cold water to stop cooking. In a large salad bowl, combine the cooked and cooled pasta, halved cherry tomatoes, crumbled tuna, sliced black olives, sliced red onion and chopped fresh parsley. Season the salad with extra virgin olive oil, lemon juice, salt and pepper to taste. Mix all ingredients well until well seasoned. Serve the wholemeal pasta salad with cherry tomatoes and fresh, colorful tuna.

BASMATI RICE WITH STEAMED VEGETABLES

Preparation time: 10 minutes

Cooking times: 20 minutes

Doses for 4 people

Ingredients

Basmati rice: 300g

Mixed vegetables (carrots, courgettes, broccoli, peas): 400g, cut into pieces Garlic: 2 cloves, finely chopped

Fresh ginger: 1 teaspoon, grated

Turmeric powder: 1 teaspoon

Fresh coriander: 2 tablespoons, finely chopped (optional)

Extra virgin olive oil: 2 tablespoons

Salt and Pepper To Taste

Preparation:

Wash the basmati rice under running water until the water becomes clear. Drain the rice well and set it aside. Prepare the vegetables, cutting them into similar sized pieces. In a steamer, bring some water to a boil. Place the vegetables in the steamer basket and cook for about 10/15 minutes, until they are tender but still crunchy. While the vegetables are cooking, heat the olive oil in a saucepan and sauté the garlic and grated ginger until golden and fragrant. Add the basmati rice to the sautéed garlic and ginger and toast for a few minutes. Add turmeric powder and mix well.

Add the hot water to the basmati rice according to the proportions indicated on the package and bring to the boil. Reduce the heat to low, cover the pan with a lid and let the rice cook for about 15/20 minutes, until it is cooked and all the liquid is absorbed. Once ready, turn off the heat and leave the basmati rice covered for a few minutes. Serve the basmati rice with the steamed vegetables, garnishing with chopped fresh coriander if desired.

SPELLED WITH COURGETTES

GRILLED MEATS AND FETA

Preparation time: 10 minutes

Cooking times: 30 minutes

Doses for 4 people

Ingredients

Pearled spelled: 300g

Courgettes: 3 medium, cut into thin rounds

Feta: 150g, cut into cubes

Cherry tomatoes: 200g, cut in half

Red onion: 1 medium, thinly sliced

Fresh parsley: 2 tablespoons, finely chopped

Extra virgin olive oil: 3 tablespoons

Lemon juice: 2 tablespoons

Salt and Pepper To Taste

Preparation:

Cook the pearled spelled in salted water following the instructions on the package, until tender but still al dente. Drain and leave to cool slightly. Meanwhile, heat a grill or non-stick pan. Grill the courgette rounds until soft and lightly browned on both sides. In a large salad bowl, combine the cooked farro, grilled zucchini, halved cherry tomatoes, sliced red onion and diced feta. Season the salad with extra virgin olive oil, lemon juice, salt and pepper to your taste. Mix all ingredients well until well seasoned. Serve the spelled.

WHOLE WHOLE LINGUINE WITH BROCCOLI AND ANCHOVIES

Preparation time: 10 minutes

Cooking times: 15 minutes

Doses for 4 people

Ingredients

Wholemeal linguine: 400g

Broccoli: 1 bunch, divided into florets

Anchovies in oil: 8 fillets,

finely chopped

Garlic: 3 cloves, finely chopped

Fresh chili pepper: 1,

finely chopped (optional)

Fresh parsley:

2 tablespoons, finely chopped

Extra virgin olive oil: 4 tablespoons

Salt to taste

Preparation:

Cook the wholemeal linguine in plenty of salted water following the instructions on the package, until al dente. In the last 5 minutes of cooking the pasta, add the broccoli florets to the linguine cooking water and cook until tender. Meanwhile, in a large pan, heat the olive oil and sauté the garlic and fresh chilli (if using) for a couple of minutes. Add the finely chopped anchovies to the pan and sauté them for a few minutes until they break down and mix with the oil. Drain the linguine and broccoli, reserving a little of the cooking water. Add the linguine and broccoli to the pan with the anchovies, adding a little pasta cooking water if necessary to create a sauce. Add salt if necessary. Serve wholemeal linguine with hot broccoli and anchovies, garnished with chopped fresh parsley.

VEGETABLE MINESTRONE WITH MIXED LEGUMES

Preparation time: 15 minutes

Cooking times: 30 minutes

Doses for 4 people

Ingredients

Courgettes: 2 medium, diced

Carrots: 2 medium, diced

Celery: 2 stalks, diced

Potatoes: 2 medium, peeled and diced

Fresh tomatoes: 4 large, diced

Onion: 1 medium, chopped

Garlic: 3 cloves, finely chopped

Canned cannellini: 400g, drained and rinsed

Vegetable broth: 1 litre

Mixed pasta (small shells, ditalini,) 100g

Extra virgin olive oil: 2 tablespoons

Salt and Pepper To Taste

Preparation:

In a large saucepan, heat the olive oil and sauté the onion and garlic until golden brown. Add the courgettes, carrots, celery and diced potatoes to the pot and cook for a few minutes until they start to soften. Add the diced fresh tomatoes and cook for another 5 minutes. Pour the vegetable broth into the pot and bring to the boil. Reduce the heat and simmer the minestrone for about 15/20 minutes or until the vegetables are tender. Add the drained cannellini beans and mixed pasta to the pot and continue to cook for another 10 minutes or until the pasta is al dente. Season with salt and pepper according to your taste. Serve the vegetable minestrone with mixed legumes hot, perhaps accompanied by croutons

QUINOA WITH TOMATOES AND FETA

Preparation time: 10 minutes

Cooking times: 15 minutes

Doses for 4 people

Ingredients

Quinoa: 1 cup (200g)

Cherry tomatoes:

200g, cut in half

Feta: 100g, crumbled

Fresh parsley:

2 tablespoons, chopped

Lemon juice: from half a lemon

Extra olive oil

virgin: 2 tbsp

Salt and Pepper To Taste

Preparation:

Rinse the quinoa well under running water. Cook the quinoa in lightly salted water following the package instructions, until it is tender and has absorbed all the water. In a large bowl, combine the cooked quinoa, halved cherry tomatoes and crumbled feta. Season with lemon juice, olive oil, chopped fresh parsley, salt and pepper to taste. Mix all ingredients well until well seasoned. Serve quinoa with cherry tomatoes and feta as a main course or side dish.

ZUCCHINI TAGLIATELLE WITH FRESH TOMATO SAUCE

Preparation time: 10 minutes

Cooking times: 10 minutes

Doses for 4 people

Ingredients

Zucchini: 4 medium

Ripe tomatoes: 4

large, cut into cubes

Garlic: 3 cloves, finely chopped

Fresh basil: 1

bunch, finely chopped

Extra olive oil

virgin: 3 tbsp

Salt and Pepper To Taste

Preparation:

Use a vegetable peeler or mandolin to cut the zucchini into thin, tagliatelle-like strips. In a pan, heat the olive oil and sauté the garlic until golden and fragrant. Add the diced ripe tomatoes to the pan and cook for about 5/7 minutes, until they become soft and form a sauce. Season with salt and pepper to taste. Add the courgette strips to the pan with the tomato sauce and sauté them for about 2/3 minutes, until heated through but still crunchy. Add the chopped fresh basil and mix well. Serve the courgette tagliatelle with fresh tomato sauce hot, possibly garnished with additional fresh basil.

PEARL BARLEY WITH ARTICHOKES AND PECORINO

Preparation time: 10 minutes

Cooking times: 20 minutes

Doses for 4 people

Ingredients

Pearl barley: 300g

Artichokes: 4 artichoke hearts,

cut into thin slices

Grated pecorino: 100g

Fresh parsley: 2 tablespoons, finely chopped

Garlic: 2 cloves, finely chopped

Vegetable broth: 750ml

Extra virgin olive oil: 3 tablespoons

Salt and Pepper To Taste

Preparation:

In a saucepan, heat the olive oil and sauté the garlic until golden and fragrant. Add the artichoke slices to the pan and brown them for a few minutes. Add the pearl barley to the pan and toast it lightly for about 2/3 minutes. Gradually add the hot vegetable broth to the pot, a ladle at a time, stirring occasionally, until the barley is cooked and has absorbed most of the liquid, which will take about 15/20 minutes. Once cooked, add salt and pepper to taste. Remove the pan from the heat and add the grated pecorino and chopped fresh parsley. Mix well until the cheese has melted and the ingredients are well combined. Serve the pearl barley with artichokes and hot pecorino, possibly garnishing with a little fresh parsley.

ZUCCHINI SPAGHETTI WITH AVOCADO PESTO

Preparation time: 15 minutes

Cooking times: 0 minutes

Doses for 4 people

Ingredients

Zucchini: 4 medium

Ripe avocado: 1 large

Fresh basil: 1 bunch

Almonds: 50g, toasted

Lemon juice: from 1 lemon

Garlic: 1 clove

Extra olive oil

virgin: 4 tbsp

Salt and Pepper To Taste

Preparation:

Use a vegetable peeler or spiralizer to cut the zucchini into spaghetti. In a food processor or blender, combine the avocado pulp, fresh basil, toasted almonds, garlic, lemon juice, olive oil, salt and pepper. Blend until you obtain a creamy consistency. In a large bowl, combine the zucchini noodles with the avocado pesto and toss gently until the zucchini is completely coated. Serve the zucchini spaghetti with avocado pesto as a main course or accompaniment.

BROWN RICE WITH ROASTED PEPPERS AND FRESH CHEESE

Preparation time: 15 minutes

Cooking times: 30 minutes

Doses for 4 people

Ingredients

Brown rice: 300g

Mixed peppers

(red, yellow, green):

3 large, cut into strips Cheese

fresh (such as mozzarella or ricotta):

200g, diced Parsley

fresh: 2 tablespoons, finely chopped

Garlic: 2 cloves, finely chopped

Vegetable broth: 600ml

Extra olive oil

virgin: 3 tbsp

Salt and Pepper To Taste

Preparation:

Preheat the oven to 200°C. Arrange the pepper strips on a baking tray lined with baking paper. Season with a drizzle of olive oil, salt and pepper. Bake in the oven for about 20/25 minutes or until the peppers are soft and lightly golden. Meanwhile, rinse the brown rice under running water and drain. In a saucepan, heat the olive oil and sauté the garlic until golden and fragrant. Add the brown rice to the pot and toast it lightly for a couple of minutes.

Add the hot vegetable broth to the pan, bring
to the boil, then reduce the heat and simmer,
covered, for about 25/30 minutes or until the
rice is cooked and has absorbed the liquid.
Once cooked, turn off the heat and let the
rice rest for a few minutes. Combine the
roasted peppers with the rice, add the diced
fresh cheese and the chopped fresh parsley.
Mix gently until the ingredients are well
combined. Serve brown rice with roasted
peppers and warm cream cheese.

WHOLEMEWHEAT PENNE WITH CAULIFLOWER AND CRISPY SPECK

Preparation time: 15 minutes

Cooking times: 20 minutes

Doses for 4 people

Ingredients

Wholemeal penne: 400g

Cauliflower: 1 medium,

divided into florets

Speck: 100g, cut into strips

Garlic: 2 cloves, finely chopped

Grated parmesan: 50g

Extra olive oil

virgin: 3 tbsp

Salt and Pepper To Taste

Preparation:

Cook the wholemeal penne in plenty of salted water following the instructions on the package, until al dente. Drain them and keep them aside. Meanwhile, in a large pan, heat a little olive oil and brown the crispy speck. Remove it from the pan and keep it aside. In the same pan, add a little more olive oil and sauté the garlic until golden and fragrant. Add the cauliflower florets to the pan and sauté for a few minutes until tender but still crunchy. Add the wholemeal penne to the pan with the cauliflower, then add the crispy speck. Season with salt and pepper to taste and mix all the ingredients well. Serve the wholemeal penne with cauliflower and crispy speck, sprinkled with freshly grated parmesan.

VENERE RICE WITH GRILLED VEGETABLES AND GREEN OLIVES

Preparation time: 15 minutes

Cooking times: 30 minutes

Doses for 4 people

Ingredients

Venere rice: 320g

Mixed vegetables for grilling

(peppers, aubergines, courgettes):

500g, cut into pieces

Pitted green olives: 100g

Cherry tomatoes: 200g, cut in half

Garlic: 3 cloves, finely chopped

Fresh basil: 1 bunch, finely chopped

Vegetable broth: 750ml

Extra virgin olive oil: 4 tablespoons

Salt and Pepper To Taste

Preparation:

Preheat a grill or grill pan over medium-high heat. Grill the mixed vegetables until tender and lightly charred, then set aside. In a saucepan, heat the olive oil and sauté the garlic until golden and fragrant. Add the Venere rice to the pan and toast it lightly for a couple of minutes. Gradually add the hot vegetable broth to the pot, one ladle at a time, stirring occasionally, until the rice is cooked and has absorbed the liquid, it will take about 25/30 minutes. Once cooked, add salt and pepper to taste. Add the grilled vegetables, pitted green olives and halved cherry tomatoes to the pot with the Venere rice. Mix gently until the ingredients are well combined. Serve the Venere rice with grilled vegetables and green olives hot, garnished with fresh chopped basil.

WHOLE WHOLE RISOTTO WITH ASPARAGUS AND PARMESAN

Preparation time: 10 minutes

Cooking times: 25 minutes

Doses for 4 people

Ingredients

Brown rice: 300g

Asparagus: 1 bunch, cut into pieces

Onion: 1 medium, finely chopped

Vegetable broth: 1 litre

Dry white wine: 125ml

Grated Parmesan: 100g

Butter: 2 tablespoons

Extra virgin olive oil: 2 tablespoons

Salt and Pepper To Taste

Preparation:

In a saucepan, bring the vegetable broth to the boil, then reduce the heat and keep it warm. In a large skillet, heat the olive oil and butter over medium heat. Add the chopped onion and fry until transparent. Add the brown rice to the pan with the onion and toast it lightly for a couple of minutes. Add the dry white wine to the rice and stir until absorbed. Begin adding the hot vegetable broth to the rice one ladle at a time, stirring occasionally and waiting for it to be absorbed before adding the next. After about 15 minutes, add the asparagus to the risotto and continue to cook until the rice is cooked, add the parmesan and serve hot.

WHOLE WHOLE PASTA WITH AUBERGINES AND DRIED TOMATOES

Preparation time: 15 minutes

Cooking times: 20 minutes

Doses for 4 people

Ingredients

Wholemeal pasta: 400g

Aubergines: 2 medium, cut into cubes

Dried tomatoes: 100g, soaked

in hot water for 10 minutes and drained

Garlic: 3 cloves, finely chopped

Fresh red chili pepper: 1 piece,

finely chopped (optional)

Fresh parsley: 2

spoons, finely chopped

Extra virgin olive oil: 4 tablespoons

Salt and Pepper To Taste

Preparation:

Cook the wholemeal pasta in plenty of salted water following the instructions on the package, until al dente. Drain it and keep it aside. In a large skillet, heat the olive oil and sauté the garlic and chilli (if using) until golden and fragrant. Add the diced aubergines to the pan and cook until soft and lightly browned. Add the soaked and drained dried tomatoes to the pan with the aubergines and cook for another 5 minutes. Season with salt and pepper to your taste. Add the wholemeal pasta to the pan with the aubergines and dried tomatoes. Mix all the ingredients well until the pasta is well seasoned. Serve the wholemeal pasta with aubergines and dried tomatoes, sprinkled with chopped fresh parsley.

SPELLED SOUP AND SEASONAL VEGETABLES

Preparation time: 15 minutes

Cooking times: 40 minutes

Doses for 4 people

Ingredients

Pearled spelled: 200g

Seasonal vegetables

(such as carrots, celery, potatoes,

courgettes): 500g, cut into cubes

Onion: 1 medium, finely chopped

Vegetable broth: 1 litre

Fresh parsley:

2 tablespoons, finely chopped

Extra virgin olive oil: 2 tablespoons

Salt and Pepper To Taste

Preparation:

In a large saucepan, heat the olive oil and sauté the onion until translucent. Add the diced seasonal vegetables to the pan and brown them for a few minutes. Add the pearled spelled to the pan with the vegetables and toast it lightly for a couple of minutes. Pour the hot vegetable broth into the pan, bring to the boil, then reduce the heat and simmer, covered, for about 30/35 minutes or until the spelled is cooked and the vegetables are soft. Season with salt and pepper to taste. Serve the spelled and seasonal vegetable soup hot, garnished with fresh chopped parsley.

WHOLE WHOLE LINGUINE WITH CLAMS AND TOMATOES

Preparation time: 15 minutes

Cooking times: 15 minutes

Doses for 4 people

Ingredients (in grams):

Wholemeal linguine: 400g

Fresh clams: 500g, shelled and cleaned

Cherry tomatoes: 200g, cut in half

Garlic: 4 cloves, finely chopped

Fresh chili pepper: 1 piece,

finely chopped (optional)

Fresh parsley: 3

spoons, finely chopped

Dry white wine: 125ml

Extra virgin olive oil: 4 tablespoons

Salt to taste

Preparation:

Cook the wholemeal linguine in plenty of salted water following the instructions on the package, until al dente. Drain them and keep them aside. In a large skillet, heat the olive oil and sauté the garlic and chilli (if using) until golden and fragrant. Add the clams to the pan and cook them over medium-high heat until they open. Add the cherry tomatoes cut in half to the pan with the clams and sauté for a few minutes. Pour in the dry white wine and let the alcohol evaporate. Add salt according to your taste. Add the wholemeal linguine to the pan with the clams and cherry tomatoes. Mix all the ingredients well until the pasta is well seasoned. Serve the wholemeal linguine with clams and cherry tomatoes, garnished with chopped fresh parsley.

WHOLE WHOLE PASTA SALAD WITH TUNA AND OLIVES

Preparation time: 15 minutes

Cooking times: 10 minutes

Doses for 4 people

Ingredients (in grams):

Short wholemeal pasta

(penne, fusilli, etc.): 400g

Tuna in oil: 200g, drained

Pitted black olives: 100g

Cherry tomatoes: 200g, cut in half

Pickled Gherkins: 4/5, sliced

Red onion: 1 small, thinly sliced

Fresh chili pepper: 1 piece, finely chopped (optional)

Fresh parsley: 3 tablespoons, finely chopped

Lemon juice: from 1 lemon

Extra virgin olive oil: 4 tablespoons

Salt and Pepper To Taste

Preparation:

Cook the wholemeal pasta in plenty of salted water following the instructions on the package, until al dente. Drain and rinse under cold water to stop cooking. In a large bowl, combine the whole-wheat pasta with the drained tuna, pitted black olives, halved cherry tomatoes, sliced pickled gherkins and sliced red onion. Add chopped fresh chili pepper (if using) and chopped fresh parsley. Season the pasta salad with lemon juice, olive oil and serve.

BLACK RICE WITH AVOCADO AND CORN

Preparation time: 15 minutes

Cooking times: 40 minutes

Doses for 4 people

Ingredients

Black rice: 320g

Ripe avocado: 2,

peeled and cut into cubes

Sweet corn: 200g, drained

Red onion: 1 medium,

finely chopped

Lime juice: from 2 limes

Fresh coriander: 4

spoons, finely chopped

Extra virgin olive oil: 3 tablespoons

Salt and Pepper To Taste

Preparation:

In a saucepan, cook the black rice according to package instructions until cooked al dente. Drain it and keep it aside. In a large bowl, combine the cooked black rice, diced avocado, and drained sweet corn. Add the chopped red onion and fresh cilantro to the rice, avocado, and corn mixture. Squeeze the lime juice over the salad and add the olive oil. Stir gently to combine all ingredients. Season with salt and pepper to your taste. Serve black rice with avocado and corn as a side or main course.

SPELLED WITH COURGETTES AND DRIED TOMATOES

Preparation time: 15 minutes

Cooking times: 30 minutes

Doses for 4 people

Ingredients

Pearled spelled: 300g

Courgettes: 3 medium, cut into cubes

Dried tomatoes: 100g, soaked in

hot water for 10 minutes and drained

Onion: 1 medium, finely chopped

Garlic: 3 cloves, finely chopped

Fresh parsley:

3 tablespoons, finely chopped

Vegetable broth: 750ml

Extra virgin olive oil: 3 tablespoons

Salt and Pepper To Taste

Preparation:

In a saucepan, bring the vegetable broth to a boil and then reduce the heat to low to keep it warm. In a large skillet, heat the olive oil and sauté the garlic and onion until golden and fragrant. Add the diced courgettes to the pan and cook until tender but still crunchy. Add the pearled spelled to the pan with the courgettes and toast it lightly for a couple of minutes. Gradually pour the hot vegetable broth into the pan, a ladle at a time, stirring occasionally, until the spelled is cooked al dente and has absorbed the liquid, it will take about 25/30 minutes. Cut the soaked dried tomatoes into strips and add them to the pan with the spelled and courgettes. Season with salt and pepper to your taste. Serve the spelled with courgettes and dried tomatoes hot, garnished with chopped fresh parsley.

RICE SPAGHETTI WITH PRAWNS AND COURGETTES

Preparation time: 15 minutes

Cooking times: 15 minutes

Doses for 4 people

Ingredients

Rice spaghetti: 400g

Shelled prawns: 300g

Zucchini: 2 medium, cut into cubes

Garlic: 3 cloves, finely chopped

Fresh chili pepper: 1 piece,

finely chopped (optional)

Fresh parsley: 3

spoons, finely chopped

Extra virgin olive oil: 4 tablespoons

Lemon juice: from 1 lemon

Salt and Pepper To Taste

Preparation:

Cook the rice spaghetti in plenty of salted water following the instructions on the package, until they are al dente. Drain them and keep them aside. In a large skillet, heat the olive oil and sauté the garlic and chilli (if using) until golden and fragrant. Add the peeled prawns to the pan and cook until pink and fully cooked. Add the diced courgettes to the pan with the prawns and cook until tender but still crunchy. Squeeze the lemon juice over the shrimp and courgettes. Add the rice noodles to the pan with the shrimp and courgettes. Mix all the ingredients well until the pasta is well seasoned. Season with salt and pepper to your taste. Serve the rice spaghetti with prawns and courgettes, garnished with chopped fresh parsley.

WHOLEMEWHEAT PENNE WITH BAKED AUBERGINES AND MOZZARELLA

Preparation time: 20 minutes

Cooking times: 30 minutes

Doses for 4 people

Ingredients

Wholemeal penne: 400g

Eggplant: 2 medium, cut into cubes

Mozzarella: 200g, cut into cubes

Peeled tomatoes: 400g, chopped

Garlic: 3 cloves, finely chopped

Fresh basil: 1 bunch,

finely chopped

Grated Parmesan: 100g

Extra virgin olive oil: 4 tablespoons

Salt and Pepper To Taste

Preparation:

Cook the wholemeal penne in plenty of salted water following the instructions on the package, until al dente. Drain them and keep them aside. Preheat the oven to 180°C. Place the aubergine cubes on a baking tray and season with olive oil, salt and pepper. Bake in the oven for about 20/25 minutes or until soft and lightly golden. In a pan, heat some olive oil and fry the garlic until golden. Add the peeled tomatoes and cook for about 10 minutes, then season with salt and pepper. Add the aubergines to the tomato sauce and mix well. Add the cooked wholemeal penne in the pan with the aubergines and sauce. Add the diced mozzarella and stir until the mozzarella begins to melt. Serve the wholemeal penne with aubergines and mozzarella.

PEARL BARLEY WITH PEPPERS AND FETA

Preparation time: 10 minutes

Cooking times: 25 minutes

Doses for 4 people

Ingredients

Pearl barley: 300g

Mixed peppers (red, yellow, green):

3 pieces, cut into cubes

Feta: 200g, cut into cubes

Red onion: 1 medium, finely chopped

Garlic: 2 cloves, finely chopped

Vegetable broth: 750ml

Fresh parsley:

3 tablespoons, finely chopped

Extra virgin olive oil: 3 tablespoons

Salt and Pepper To Taste

Preparation:

In a saucepan, bring the vegetable broth to a boil and then reduce the heat to low to keep it warm. In a large skillet, heat the olive oil and sauté the garlic and onion until golden and fragrant. Add the diced peppers to the pan and cook until soft but still crunchy. Add the pearl barley to the pan with the peppers and toast it lightly for a couple of minutes. Gradually pour the hot vegetable broth into the pan, a ladle at a time, stirring occasionally, until the barley is cooked al dente and has absorbed the liquid, it will take about 20/25 minutes. Once the orzo is cooked, add the diced feta and chopped fresh parsley. Mix all the ingredients well. Season with salt and pepper to your taste. Serve pearl barley with peppers and feta hot.

BROWN RICE WITH PEAS AND RAW HAM

Preparation time: 10 minutes

Cooking times: 25 minutes

Doses for 4 people

Ingredients

Brown rice: 320g

Fresh or frozen peas: 200g

Raw ham: 100g,

cut into thin strips

Onion: 1 medium, finely chopped

Vegetable broth: 750ml

Fresh parsley:

3 tablespoons, finely chopped

Butter: 2 tablespoons

Extra virgin olive oil: 2 tablespoons

Salt and Pepper To Taste

Preparation:

In a saucepan, bring the vegetable broth to a boil and then reduce the heat to low to keep it warm. In a pan, melt the butter with the olive oil and fry the onion until transparent. Add the brown rice to the pan with the onion and toast it lightly for a couple of minutes. Gradually pour the hot vegetable broth into the pan, a ladle at a time, stirring occasionally, until the rice is cooked al dente and has absorbed the liquid, it will take about 20/25 minutes. Add fresh or frozen peas to the pan with the rice for the last 5 minutes of cooking. Once the rice is cooked, add the strips of raw ham and the chopped fresh parsley. Mix all the ingredients well. Season with salt and pepper to your taste. Serve the brown rice with peas and raw ham.

CARROT TAGLIATELLE WITH ALMOND PESTO

Preparation time: 15 minutes

Cooking times: 10 minutes

Doses for 4 people

Ingredients

Carrot tagliatelle: 400g

Almonds: 100g, toasted

Fresh basil: 1 bunch

Garlic: 2 cloves

Grated parmesan: 50g

Extra olive oil

virgin: 4 tbsp

Salt and Pepper To Taste

Preparation:

Cook the carrot tagliatelle in plenty of salted water following the instructions on the package, until al dente. Drain them and keep them aside. Meanwhile, prepare the almond pesto. In a blender, combine the toasted almonds, fresh basil, garlic, grated Parmesan and olive oil. Blend until you obtain a smooth consistency. Season with salt and pepper to taste. Season the carrot tagliatelle with the prepared almond pesto. Mix well to evenly distribute the pesto over the tagliatelle. Serve the carrot tagliatelle with hot almond pesto, garnished with chopped almonds and fresh basil leaves.

SPELLED WITH CHICKPEAS AND TOMATOES

Preparation time: 10 minutes

Cooking times: 30 minutes

Doses for 4 people

Ingredients

Spelled: 300g

Cooked chickpeas: 400g,

drained and rinsed

Cherry tomatoes:

250g, cut in half

Red onion: 1 medium,, sliced thinly

Garlic: 2 cloves, finely chopped

Fresh parsley:

3 tablespoons, finely chopped

Vegetable broth: 750ml

Extra virgin olive oil: 3 tablespoons

Salt and Pepper To Taste

Preparation:

In a saucepan, bring the vegetable broth to a boil and then reduce the heat to low to keep it warm. In a pan, heat the olive oil and sauté the garlic and red onion until golden and fragrant. Add the halved cherry tomatoes to the pan with the garlic and onion and cook until slightly softened. Add the cooked chickpeas to the pan with the cherry tomatoes and mix well. Add the spelled to the pan with the cherry tomatoes and chickpeas. Gradually pour the hot vegetable broth into the pan, one ladle at a time, stirring occasionally, until the spelled is cooked al dente and has absorbed the liquid, it will take about 25/30 minutes. Season with salt and pepper to your taste. Serve the spelled with chickpeas and cherry tomatoes hot, garnished with fresh chopped parsley.

RECIPES
SECOND DISHES

GRILLED SALMON WITH STEAMED ASPARAGUS

Preparation time: 10 minutes

Cooking times: 15 minutes

Doses for 4 people

Ingredients

Salmon: 4 fillets,

approximately 150g each

Asparagus: 500g,

washed and chopped

Extra olive oil

virgin: 4 tbsp

Lemon juice: from 1 lemon

Salt and Pepper To Taste

Preparation:

Preheat grill to medium-high heat.

Season the salmon fillets with olive oil, lemon juice, salt and pepper. Grill the salmon for about 5/7 minutes per side or until cooked. Meanwhile, prepare the steamed asparagus. Place the asparagus in a steamer and cook for approximately 5/7 minutes or until tender but still crunchy. Season the asparagus with a drizzle of olive oil, salt and pepper. Serve the grilled salmon with steamed asparagus as a side dish.

GRILLED CHICKEN WITH ARTICHOKES AND ROASTED PEPPERS

Preparation time: 20 minutes

Cooking times: 25 minutes

Doses for 4 people

Ingredients

Chicken breast: 4 pieces, cut into thin slices

Artichokes: 4 artichoke hearts, cleaned and cut into slices

Red and yellow peppers: 2 pieces, cut into strips

Extra virgin olive oil: 4 tablespoons

Lemon juice: from 1 lemon

Garlic: 3 cloves, finely chopped

Fresh rosemary:

2 sprigs, finely chopped

Salt and Pepper To Taste

Preparation:

Preheat grill to medium-high heat. Season the chicken breast slices with olive oil, lemon juice, garlic, rosemary, salt and pepper. Grill the chicken for about 5 to 6 minutes per side or until cooked through. While the chicken cooks, grill the artichoke hearts and bell pepper strips until tender and lightly browned. Season the artichokes and peppers with a drizzle of olive oil, lemon juice, salt and pepper. Serve the grilled chicken with artichokes and roasted peppers on the side.

SHRIMP AND MIXED VEGETABLES SKEWERS

Preparation time: 20 minutes

Cooking times: 10 minutes

Doses for 4 people

Ingredients:

Large prawns, peeled

and cleaned: 16 pieces

Zucchini: 2 medium, chopped

in thick washers

Peppers (red, green, yellow):

2, cut into cubes

Red onions: 1 large,

cut into wedges

Cherry tomatoes: 16, whole

Extra virgin olive oil: 4 tablespoons

Lemon juice: 2 tablespoons

Salt and Pepper To Taste

Preparation:

Preheat grill or barbecue to medium-high heat. Thread the prawns and vegetables alternately onto skewers. Brush the skewers with olive oil and lemon juice and season with salt and pepper. Cook the skewers on the heated grill for about 3 to 4 minutes per side or until the shrimp are pink and the vegetables are tender. Serve hot and enjoy the delicious skewers of prawns and mixed vegetables.

PORK CHOPS WITH ARTICHOKES AND BAKED POTATOES

Preparation time: 20 minutes

Cooking times: 1 hour

Doses for 4 people

Ingredients:

Pork chops: 4 pieces (150g each)

Artichokes: 4 hearts, cleaned and cut into slices

Potatoes: 4 medium, peeled

and cut into slices

Garlic: 4 cloves, finely chopped

Fresh rosemary: 2 sprigs,

finely chopped

Chicken broth: 1 cup

Extra virgin olive oil: 4 tablespoons

Salt and Pepper To Taste

Preparation:

Preheat the oven to 180°C. Make incisions on the pork chops and season them with salt, pepper, garlic and rosemary. Arrange the artichoke and potato slices on a baking sheet and place the pork chops on top of the vegetables. Pour the chicken broth into the roasting pan and drizzle with olive oil. Cover the pan with foil and bake in the preheated oven for about 45 minutes. Remove the foil and continue to cook for another 15 to 20 minutes or until the pork chops are browned and tender. Serve hot pork chops with artichokes and baked potatoes.

COD IN PAPER WITH ASPARAGUS AND TOMATOES

Preparation time: 15 minutes

Cooking times: 20 minutes

Doses for 4 people

Ingredients:

Cod fillets:

4 pieces (200g each)

Asparagus: 12, cleaned

and cut into pieces

Cherry tomatoes:

200g, cut in half

Garlic: 2 cloves, finely chopped

Fresh parsley:

2 tablespoons, finely chopped

Extra virgin olive oil: 4 tablespoons

Lemon juice: 2 tablespoons

Salt and Pepper To Taste

Preparation:

Preheat the oven to 200°C. Cut 4 sheets of baking paper, one for each cod fillet. Distribute the asparagus and cherry tomatoes on each sheet of baking paper. Place a cod fillet on each bed of vegetables. Season the fish and vegetables with minced garlic, fresh parsley, olive oil, lemon juice, salt and pepper. Close the parcels, forming well-sealed envelopes. Place the parcels on a baking tray and bake for about 15/20 minutes or until the fish is cooked and the vegetables are tender. Serve the cod in foil hot directly in their packages.

ARTICHOKE AND SPINACH OMELETTE

Preparation time: 15 minutes

Cooking times: 15 minutes

Doses for 4 people

Ingredients:

Eggs: 6

Artichokes: 2, cleaned and

cut into thin slices

Fresh spinach: 200g, washed and chopped

Onion: 1 medium, finely chopped

Grated cheese: 50g

(pecorino or parmesan)

Extra virgin olive oil: 2 tablespoons

Salt and Pepper To Taste

Preparation:

In a non-stick pan, heat the olive oil and fry the onion until transparent. Add the sliced artichokes and cook until they become soft. Add the chopped spinach and cook until wilted and releasing its liquid. In a bowl, beat the eggs with the grated cheese, salt and pepper. Pour the egg mixture over the vegetables in the pan. Cook over medium-low heat for about 10/15 minutes or until the omelette is cooked and golden on the edges. Use a spatula to lift the edges of the omelet and allow the uncooked liquid to flow underneath them. Once cooked, slide the omelette onto a serving plate and cut it into wedges before serving.

BEEF FILLET WITH PAN-SAUTEED ASPARAGUS

Preparation time: 10 minutes

Cooking times: 15 minutes

Doses for 4 people

Ingredients:

Beef fillet: 4 pieces,

(about 150g each)

Asparagus: 400g,

washed and cut into pieces

Garlic: 2 cloves, finely chopped

Extra virgin olive oil: 4 tablespoons

Lemon juice: 2 tablespoons

Salt and Pepper To Taste

Preparation:

Heat a non-stick pan over medium-high heat. Season the beef fillets with salt, pepper and lemon juice. Add two tablespoons of olive oil to the pan and heat. Cook the beef tenderloins in the pan for about 3 to 4 minutes per side for medium rare or until they reach the desired doneness. Remove from pan and let rest. In the same pan, add two more tablespoons of olive oil and the minced garlic. Add the cut asparagus to the pan and sauté for about 5/7 minutes or until tender but still crunchy. Season the asparagus with salt and pepper to taste. Serve the beef fillets with the pan-fried asparagus as a side dish.

BAKED SOLE WITH ARTICHOKES AND OLIVES

Preparation time: 15 minutes

Cooking times: 20 minutes

Doses for 4 people

Ingredients:

Sole: 4 fillets (about 200g each)

Artichokes: 4 hearts, cleaned and cut into slices

Black olives: 1/2 cup,

pitted and cut into rounds

Garlic: 3 cloves, finely chopped,

Fresh parsley:

2 tablespoons, finely chopped

Dry white wine: 1/4 cup

Extra virgin olive oil: 4 tablespoons

Salt and pepper to taste 6.

Preparation:

Preheat the oven to 180°C. In a pan, heat two tablespoons of olive oil and add the chopped garlic cloves and sliced artichokes. Cook until the artichokes are soft. Add the pitted olives and chopped fresh parsley, then blend with the white wine. Let the alcohol evaporate. Place the sole fillets on a baking tray lightly greased with olive oil. Season with salt and pepper. Pour the artichoke, olive and wine mixture over the fillets. Cover the pan with foil and bake for about 15/20 minutes, or until the sole is cooked and flakes easily with a fork. Serve the baked sole with artichokes and olives hot, accompanied by a side dish of your choice.

CHICKEN ROLLS WITH ASPARAGUS AND CHEESE

Preparation time: 20 minutes

Cooking times: 25 minutes

Doses for 4 people

Ingredients:

Chicken breast: 4 thin slices

Asparagus: 16 tips,

clean and blanched

Sliced cheese (type

provola or fontina): 4 slices

Extra olive oil

virgin: 4 tbsp

Salt and Pepper To Taste

Preparation:

Preheat the oven to 180°C. Place a slice of cheese on each slice of chicken breast. Add 4 asparagus tips to each cheese slice. Roll the chicken breast slices around the asparagus and cheese to form the rolls. Secure the rolls with toothpicks. Heat the olive oil in a nonstick skillet over medium-high heat. Brown the chicken rolls on all sides until golden brown. Transfer the rolls to a baking tray and bake for about 15 to 20 minutes or until the chicken is cooked through. Remove toothpicks before serving. You can add salt and pepper to taste before serving.

MIXED GRILLED VEGETABLES WITH CHICKEN BREAST

Preparation time: 20 minutes

Cooking times: 15 minutes

Doses for 4 people

Ingredients:

Chicken breast: 4 fillets

Courgettes: 2, cut into long slices

Peppers (red, yellow, green):

2, cut into strips

Eggplant: 1, sliced

Mushrooms: 200g, cut into slices

Extra virgin olive oil: 4 tablespoons

Garlic: 2 cloves, finely chopped

Fresh parsley:

2 tablespoons, finely chopped

Salt and Pepper To Taste

 Preparation:

Heat a grill or grill pan over medium-high heat. Season the chicken breast fillets with olive oil, minced garlic, parsley, salt and pepper. Grill the chicken fillets for about 6 to 8 minutes per side or until they are cooked through and have nice streaks. In the meantime, also grill the vegetables seasoned with olive oil, salt and pepper for about 4/5 minutes per side or until they are tender and lightly golden. Serve grilled chicken breasts with grilled mixed vegetables as a side dish.

COD WITH ARTICHOKES AND TOMATOES

Preparation time: 20 minutes

Cooking times: 25 minutes

Doses for 4 people

Ingredients:

Cod fillets: 4 pieces,

soaked and cleaned (about 200g each)

Artichokes: 4 hearts, cleaned and cut into wedges

Cherry tomatoes: 200g, cut in half

Garlic: 3 cloves, finely chopped

Fresh parsley:

2 tablespoons, finely chopped

Dry white wine: 1/4 cup

Extra virgin olive oil: 4 tablespoons

Salt and Pepper To Taste

Preparation:

In a large skillet, heat two tablespoons of olive oil and add the minced garlic cloves. Add the chopped artichoke hearts and cherry tomatoes. Cook over medium-low heat until the artichokes become soft and the cherry tomatoes begin to release their juices. Add the white wine and let the alcohol evaporate. In another pan, heat the remaining two tablespoons of olive oil and cook the cod fillets on both sides until golden. Add the cod fillets to the pan with the artichokes and cherry tomatoes. Sprinkle with chopped fresh parsley and season with salt and pepper. Continue cooking over medium heat for another 5 to 7 minutes, or until the fish is fully cooked and the vegetables are tender. Serve the cod with artichokes and cherry tomatoes hot, accompanied by crunchy bread or a side dish of your choice.

VEAL SCALLOPPINE WITH ASPARAGUS AND LEMON

Preparation time: 15 minutes

Cooking times: 15 minutes

Doses for 4 people

Ingredients:

Veal scallops: 8 pieces, thin

Asparagus: 20 tips,

clean and cut in half

Lemon: 1, juice and

grated zest

Beef broth: 1/2 cup

Flour: 4 tablespoons

Butter: 4 tablespoons

Salt and Pepper To Taste

Preparation:

Salt and pepper the veal escalopes and dredge them in the flour. In a large skillet, melt the butter over medium-high heat. Add the veal escalopes and cook them for 2/3 minutes on each side, or until they are golden. Remove the scallops from the pan and set aside. In the same pan, add the asparagus tips and sauté them for 3/4 minutes, until tender. Add the lemon juice and grated zest and the meat broth. Place the scallops back in the pan and cook them for another 2/3 minutes, so that they become flavorful with the sauce. Serve the veal escalopes with the hot asparagus and lemon sauce.

SALMON IN ALMOND CRUST WITH STEAMED ARTICHOKES

Preparation time: 15 minutes

Cooking times: 20 minutes

Doses for 4 people

Ingredients:

Salmon fillets: 4 pieces

(about 200g each)

Chopped almonds: 1/2 cup

Fresh parsley:

2 tablespoons, finely chopped

Grated lemon zest: from 1 lemon

Extra virgin olive oil: 4 tablespoons

Artichokes: 4, cleaned and cut into slices

Lemon juice: from 1 lemon

Salt and Pepper To Taste

Preparation:

Preheat the oven to 200°C. In a bowl, mix the chopped almonds, chopped fresh parsley and grated lemon zest. Lightly coat the salmon fillets with a little olive oil. Sprinkle the almond crust evenly over the salmon fillets. Place the salmon fillets on a baking tray lined with baking paper. Bake in the oven for about 12/15 minutes or until the salmon is cooked and the crust is golden. Meanwhile, bring a pot of lightly salted water to a boil. Add the sliced artichokes and steam for about 8/10 minutes or until tender. Drain them and season them with lemon juice, salt and pepper. Serve the almond crusted salmon with the steamed artichokes as a side dish.

MIXED MEATBALLS WITH COURGETTES AND CARROTS

Preparation time: 20 minutes

Cooking times: 25 minutes

Doses for 4 people

Ingredients:

Mixed minced meat

(beef and pork): 500g

Courgettes: 2 medium, grated

Carrots: 2 medium, grated

Eggs: 2

Breadcrumbs: 1/2 cup

Grated cheese: 1/4 cup

Fresh parsley:

2 tablespoons, finely chopped

Garlic: 2 cloves, finely chopped

Salt and Pepper To Taste

Extra virgin olive oil:

to grease the pan

Preparation:

Preheat the oven to 200°C and lightly grease a baking tray with olive oil. In a large bowl, combine the ground beef, grated zucchini, grated carrots, eggs, breadcrumbs, grated cheese, chopped fresh parsley, minced garlic, salt and pepper. Shape meatballs with your hands and place them on the prepared baking sheet. Bake in the preheated oven for about 20/25 minutes or until the meatballs are golden brown and fully cooked. Serve the mixed meatballs with hot courgettes and carrots as a main course or side dish, as desired.

GRILLED SWORDFISH WITH ASPARAGUS AND LEMON SAUCE

Preparation time: 15 minutes

Cooking times: 10/12 minutes

Doses for 4 people

Ingredients:

Swordfish fillets: 4 pieces

(about 200g each)

Asparagus: 1 bunch,

cleaned and cut in half

Lemon: 2, one for juice

and one sliced to decorate

Extra olive oil

virgin: 4 tbsp

Salt and Pepper To Taste

Preparation:

Preheat grill to medium-high heat. Brush the swordfish fillets with olive oil, lemon juice, salt and pepper. Grill the swordfish for about 4/6 minutes per side, or until it is cooked and slightly golden. While the swordfish cooks, grill the asparagus with a little olive oil, salt and pepper until tender and slightly charred, about 6 to 8 minutes. Make the lemon sauce by mixing the remaining lemon juice with a little olive oil, salt and pepper, to your taste. Once ready, serve the grilled swordfish with asparagus and lemon sauce. You can decorate with lemon slices and fresh parsley if you wish.

ROAST PORK WITH ARTICHOKES AND SWEET POTATOES

Preparation time: 20 minutes

Cooking times: 1 hour and 30 minutes

Doses for 4 people

Ingredients:

Roast pork: 1 kg

Artichokes: 4, cleaned

and cut into segments

Sweet potatoes: 3 medium,

peeled and cut into pieces

Garlic: 4 cloves, finely chopped

Fresh rosemary: 2 sprigs

Chicken broth: 1 cup

Extra virgin olive oil: 4 tablespoons

Salt and Pepper To Taste

Preparation:

Preheat the oven to 180°C. Make shallow cuts on the surface of the pork roast and insert the garlic cloves and rosemary sprigs. Brush the pork roast with olive oil and season with salt and pepper. Place the pork roast on a baking tray and arrange the artichoke segments and sweet potatoes around it. Pour the chicken broth into the roasting pan. Cover the pan with foil and bake in the oven for about 1 hour. Remove the foil and cook for an additional 30 minutes or until the pork is browned and cooked through. Once done, let the pork roast rest for a few minutes before slicing. Serve the roast pork with the artichokes and sweet potatoes on the side.

SLICED BEEF WITH ARUGULA AND TOMATOES

Preparation time: 15 minutes

Cooking times: 10/15 minutes

Doses for 4 people

Ingredients:

Beef (per cut):

4 pieces, about 200g each

Arugula: 100g

Cherry tomatoes:

200g, cut in half

50g Parmesan, grated

Extra olive oil

virgin: 4 tbsp

Lemon juice: from 1 lemon

Salt and Pepper To Taste

Preparation:

Preheat grill or nonstick skillet over medium-high heat. Season the beef pieces with salt, pepper and a drizzle of olive oil. Grill the pieces of beef for about 3/5 minutes per side, depending on the thickness and desired degree of doneness. While the beef cooks, in a large bowl, mix the arugula with the halved cherry tomatoes. Season the arugula and cherry tomatoes with olive oil, lemon juice, salt and pepper. Once the meat is cooked, let it rest for a few minutes before slicing it. Slice the beef and arrange the slices on a bed of Arugula and cherry tomatoes. Complete with a generous sprinkling of grated parmesan. Serve the sliced beef with Arugula and cherry tomatoes hot, accompanied by crusty bread if desired.

SEA BASS IN PAPER WITH ASPARAGUS AND OLIVES

Preparation time: 15 minutes

Cooking times: 20/25 minutes

Doses for 4 people

Ingredients:

Whole sea bass: 2 (about 500g

each), clean and scaled

Asparagus: 1 bunch, cleaned and cut into pieces

Black olives: 1/2 cup, pitted

Cherry tomatoes: 200g, cut in half

Garlic: 4 cloves, finely chopped

Fresh parsley: 2

spoons, finely chopped

Dry white wine: 1/4 cup

Extra virgin olive oil: 4 tablespoons

Salt and Pepper To Taste

Preparation:

Preheat the oven to 200°C. Cut two large sheets of baking paper and place a sea bass on each. Fill the inside of each sea bass with asparagus, olives, cherry tomatoes, garlic and parsley. Season the inside and outside of the sea bass with salt, pepper, a drizzle of olive oil and a little white wine. Close the parcels, sealing them well. Place the parcels on a baking tray and cook in the preheated oven for about 20/25 minutes, or until the sea bass is cooked and the vegetables are tender. Once ready, gently open the foil and serve the sea bass cooked in foil with asparagus and olives directly on the baking paper.

TURKEY BREAST WITH ARTICHOKES AND DRIED TOMATOES

Preparation time: 15 minutes

Cooking times: 25/30 minutes

Doses for 4 people

Ingredients:

Turkey breast: 4 thin slices

Artichokes: 4 hearts of artichoke, cut into wedges

Dried tomatoes: 1/2 cup, cut into thin strips

Chicken broth: 1 cup

Garlic: 2 cloves, finely chopped

Fresh thyme: 1 tablespoon, finely chopped

Extra virgin olive oil: 4 tablespoons

Salt and Pepper To Taste

Preparation:

Preheat the oven to 180°C. In a pan, heat some olive oil and add the minced garlic. Add the artichoke hearts and dried tomatoes and sauté for a few minutes. Add the chicken broth and cook over medium heat for about 5/7 minutes, until the artichokes are tender. Meanwhile, season the turkey breast slices with salt, pepper and fresh thyme. Place the turkey breast slices on a lightly greased baking tray. Distribute the artichokes, dried tomatoes and cooking broth evenly over the turkey breast. Cover the roasting pan with aluminum foil and cook in the oven for about 20 to 25 minutes, or until the turkey is cooked and tender. Serve the turkey breast with artichokes and dried tomatoes hot, accompanied by side dishes of your choice.

STEAMED FISH WITH CRISPY VEGETABLES

Preparation time: 20 minutes

Cooking times: 15 minutes

Doses for 4 people

Ingredients:

Fish fillets of your choice: 4 pieces

(salmon, sea bass, sole, etc.)

Asparagus: 1 bunch, cleaned and cut into pieces

Carrots: 2 medium, peeled

and cut into thin sticks

Courgettes: 2 medium, cut into thin sticks

Celery: 2 stalks, cut into thin sticks

Soy sauce: 2 tablespoons

Fresh ginger: 1 tablespoon, grated

Lemon juice: from 1 lemon

Sesame oil: 1 tbsp

Salt and Pepper To Taste

Preparation:

In a steamer, bring water to a boil. Season the fish fillets with salt, pepper, lemon juice and grated ginger. Place the fish fillets and prepared vegetables on the steaming tray. Place the tray in the steamer and cover with the lid. Steam cook for about 10/12 minutes, or until the fish is cooked and the vegetables are tender but crunchy. Meanwhile, prepare the sauce by mixing the soy sauce and sesame oil. Once ready, serve the steamed fish with the crunchy vegetables, accompanied by soy sauce and sesame oil.

PIZZAIOLA-STYLE WITH ASPARAGUS AND PEPPERS

Preparation time: 15 minutes

Cooking times: 25/30 minutes

Doses for 4 people

Ingredients:

Slices of veal:

4 pieces, about 150g each

Peeled tomatoes: 400g, crushed

Peppers: 2 large, cut into strips

Asparagus: 200g, cleaned and cut into pieces

Onion: 1 large, sliced

Garlic: 3 cloves, finely chopped

Dried oregano: 1 teaspoon

Extra virgin olive oil: 4 tablespoons

Salt and Pepper To Taste

Preparation:

Preheat the oven to 180°C. Heat the olive oil in a large pan and fry the garlic and onion until golden. Add the peppers and asparagus and cook for about 5 minutes. Add the crushed peeled tomatoes, oregano, salt and pepper. Mix well and leave to cook over medium-low heat for another 10 minutes. Meanwhile, season the slices of meat with salt and pepper. Place the slices of meat on a lightly greased baking tray. Pour over the tomato sauce with peppers and asparagus. Cover the pan with aluminum foil and cook in the oven for about 20 to 25 minutes, or until the meat is cooked and tender. Once ready, serve the meat pizzaiola with asparagus and peppers hot, accompanied by side dishes of your choice.

TUNA SLICE WITH ASPARAGUS AND CITRUS SAUCE

Preparation time: 15 minutes

Cooking times: 10/12 minutes

Doses for 4 people

Ingredients:

Fresh tuna steaks: 4 pieces,

approximately 150g each

Asparagus: 1 bunch, cleaned and cut into pieces

Grated lemon zest: from 1 lemon

Orange juice: from 2 oranges

Lemon juice: from 1 lemon

Fresh ginger: 1 teaspoon, grated

Garlic: 2 cloves, finely chopped

Extra virgin olive oil: 4 tablespoons

Salt and Pepper To Taste

Preparation:

In a bowl, mix the orange juice, lemon juice, grated lemon zest, grated ginger, minced garlic, salt and pepper. Place the tuna steaks in the marinade and leave to marinate in the refrigerator for at least 30 minutes. Heat the olive oil in a non-stick pan and add the asparagus. Cook for about 5 minutes until tender but crunchy. Add the marinated tuna steaks and cook for about 2/3 minutes per side, or until the tuna is cooked but still pink inside. Once cooked, serve the tuna steak with asparagus and hot citrus sauce, accompanied by rice or potatoes to taste.

CHICKEN CURRY WITH ASPARAGUS AND PEPPERS

Preparation time: 15 minutes

Cooking times: 25/30 minutes

Doses for 4 people

Ingredients:

Chicken breast: 4 fillets, approximately

150g each cut into cubes

Asparagus: 150 g cleaned and cut into pieces

Peppers: 2 large, cut into strips

Onion: 1 large, sliced

Garlic: 3 cloves, finely chopped

Turmeric powder: 1 teaspoon

Curry powder: 2 teaspoons

Coconut milk: 1 can (400 ml)

Chicken broth: 1 cup

Extra virgin olive oil: 4 tablespoons

Salt and Pepper To Taste

Preparation:

Heat the olive oil in a large skillet over medium heat. Add the garlic and onion and sauté until golden. Add the peppers and asparagus and cook for about 5 minutes. Add the chicken cubes and cook until golden. Add the turmeric and curry powder, mix well to distribute the spices evenly. Pour the chicken broth and coconut milk into the pan. Bring to the boil, reduce the heat and simmer for about 15 to 20 minutes, or until the chicken is cooked and the vegetables are tender. Adjust salt and pepper according to taste. Serve the chicken curry with asparagus and peppers hot, accompanied by basmati rice.

BAKED TROUT WITH ARTICHOKES AND CAPERS

Preparation time: 15 minutes

Cooking times: 20/25 minutes

Doses for 4 people

Ingredients:

Whole trout: 4, cleaned and scaled

Artichokes: 4 hearts of

artichoke, cut into wedges

Capers: 4 tablespoons, rinsed

Lemon: 1, cut into thin slices

Fresh parsley:

4 tablespoons, finely chopped

Garlic: 4 cloves, finely chopped

Dry white wine: 1/2 cup

Extra virgin olive oil: 4 tablespoons

Salt and Pepper To Taste

Preparation:

Preheat the oven to 200°C. Make cuts on the side of the trout and insert lemon slices and capers into the cuts. In a bowl, mix the minced garlic, fresh parsley, salt and pepper. Stuff the trout with this garlic and parsley mixture. Arrange the artichoke hearts around the trout on the baking tray. Pour the dry white wine over the fish and artichokes. Sprinkle everything with a drizzle of extra virgin olive oil. Bake for about 20/25 minutes, or until the fish is cooked and the vegetables are tender. Once ready, serve the baked trout with artichokes and capers hot, accompanied by side dishes of your choice.

ASPARAGUS AND BACON OMELETTE

Preparation time: 10 minutes

Cooking times: 15 minutes

Doses for 4 people

Ingredients:

Eggs: 8

Asparagus: 150 g cleaned

and cut into pieces

Bacon: 100g, cut into cubes

Grated cheese (Parmesan

or Pecorino): 1/2 cup

Onion: 1, chopped

Fresh parsley:

2 tablespoons, finely chopped

Extra virgin olive oil: 2 tablespoons

Salt and Pepper To Taste

Preparation:

In a non-stick pan, heat the olive oil and add the bacon and onion. Saute until the bacon is crispy and the onion is translucent. Add the asparagus and cook for about 5/7 minutes, until they become soft. In a bowl, beat the eggs with the grated cheese, fresh parsley, salt and pepper. Pour the egg mixture over the asparagus and bacon in the skillet. Cook over medium-low heat for about 10 minutes, or until the eggs are completely set. When the omelette is ready, slide onto a serving plate and serve hot or at room temperature. Cut into wedges and serve.

SLICED BEEF WITH ARTICHOKES AND BALSAMIC VINEGAR SAUCE

Preparation time: 15 minutes

Cooking times: 15 minutes

Doses for 4 people

Ingredients:

Beef slices (sliced, sirloin):

4 pieces, about 150g each

Artichokes: 4 artichoke hearts, cut into wedges

Balsamic vinegar: 4 tablespoons

Beef broth: 1/2 cup

Garlic: 2 cloves, finely chopped

Fresh rosemary: 2

sprigs, finely chopped

Extra virgin olive oil: 4 tablespoons

Salt and Pepper To Taste

Preparation:

Heat the olive oil in a non-stick pan. Add the chopped garlic and brown it lightly. Add the beef slices and cook for approximately 3/4 minutes per side, or until the desired degree of doneness is reached. Salt and pepper to taste. Remove the beef slices from the pan and set aside. In the same pan, add the artichoke hearts and sauté for about 5 minutes, until soft. Add the beef stock and balsamic vinegar to the pan and cook for about 2 to 3 minutes, until the liquid reduces slightly. Add the fresh rosemary and season with salt and pepper to taste. Serve the slices of beef with the artichokes and balsamic vinegar sauce hot, accompanied by side dishes of your choice.

SHRIMP AND ASPARAGUS SKEWERS AND WRAPPED IN HAM

Preparation time: 15 minutes

Cooking times: 8/10 minutes

Doses for 4 people

Ingredients:

Fresh prawns: 16, peeled and cleaned

Asparagus: 16 tips

Raw ham slices: 8, cut

in half to get 16 stripes

Extra virgin olive oil: 2 tablespoons

Lemon juice: 2 tablespoons

Salt and Pepper To Taste

Preparation:

Preheat the oven grill or barbecue. Wrap each asparagus tip with a strip of ham. Thread 4 asparagus tips wrapped in ham and 4 prawns on each skewer, alternating them. Place the skewers on a baking tray lined with baking paper. Season the skewers with olive oil, lemon juice, salt and pepper. Cook the skewers in the oven grill or on the barbecue for about 8/10 minutes, turning them halfway through cooking, until the prawns are pink and the asparagus are tender. Once cooked, serve the prawn and asparagus skewers hot, accompanied by a sauce of your choice or fresh side dishes.

SALT CRUSTED SEA BASS IN WITH ARTICHOKES AND GINGER

Preparation time: 20 minutes

Cooking times: 30/35 minutes

Doses for 4 people

Ingredients:

2 whole sea bass, cleaned

Coarse salt: 2 kg

Artichokes: 4 artichoke hearts, cut into quarters

Fresh ginger: 2 tablespoons, grated

Lemon: 1, cut into thin slices

Fresh parsley: 4 tablespoons, finely chopped

Garlic: 4 cloves, finely chopped

Extra virgin olive oil: 4 tablespoons

Salt and Pepper To Taste

Preparation:

Preheat the oven to 200°C. In a bowl, mix the coarse salt with the water until you get a sandy consistency. Fill the belly of the sea bass with lemon slices, grated ginger, chopped garlic and parsley. Place half of the salt mixture on a baking sheet and place the sea bass on top. Cover the sea bass with the rest of the salt, pressing lightly to form an even crust. Bake in the oven for about 30/35 minutes, or until the salt crust becomes hard and golden. Meanwhile, in a pan, heat the olive oil and sauté the artichoke quarters with grated ginger and minced garlic for about 10/15 minutes, or until soft and golden. Serve the sea bass in a hot salt crust, accompanied by the artichokes and seasoned with extra virgin olive oil and fresh parsley.

VEAL CUTLETS WITH ASPARAGUS AND LEMON

Preparation time: 15 minutes

Cooking times: 15/20 minutes

Doses for 4 people

Ingredients:

Veal cutlets: 4 pieces

approximately 200g each

Asparagus: 1 bunch,

cleaned and cut into pieces

Lemon: 1, cut into thin slices

Flour: to taste, Eggs: 2, beaten

Breadcrumbs: to taste

Butter: 4 tablespoons

Extra virgin olive oil: 2 tablespoons

Salt and Pepper To Taste

Preparation:

Prepare three dishes: one with the flour, one with the beaten eggs and one with the breadcrumbs. Dip the veal cutlets first in the flour, then in the beaten eggs and finally in the breadcrumbs, making sure to cover them evenly. Heat the butter and olive oil in a nonstick skillet over medium-high heat. Add the breaded cutlets and cook for about 5/7 minutes per side, or until golden and evenly cooked. During the last 2 minutes of cooking, add the asparagus and lemon slices to the pan around the cutlets and cook until the asparagus is tender and the lemon is lightly caramelized. Adjust salt and pepper according to taste. Once ready, serve the veal cutlets with hot asparagus and lemon, accompanied by side dishes of your choice.

PERCH WITH ARTICHOKES AND BLACK OLIVES

Preparation time: 15 minutes

Cooking times: 20/25 minutes

Doses for 4 people

Ingredients:

Perch fillets: 4 pieces

approximately 150g each

Artichokes: 4 artichoke hearts, cut into wedges

Black olives: 1/2 cup, pitted

Peeled tomatoes: 400g, diced

Garlic: 3 cloves, finely chopped

Dry white wine: 1 glass

Fresh parsley:

4 tablespoons, finely chopped

Extra virgin olive oil: 4 tablespoons

Salt and Pepper To Taste

Preparation:

Preheat the oven to 180°C. In a pan, heat the olive oil and add the minced garlic. Brown lightly. Add the artichokes and cook them for about 5 minutes, until they are lightly golden. Add the black olives and peeled tomatoes. Mix well. Add the dry white wine and cook for another 5 minutes. Arrange the perch fillets in a baking pan and sprinkle them with the artichoke, olive and tomato mixture. Bake in the preheated oven for about 15 to 20 minutes, or until the fish is cooked through and flakes easily with a fork. Before serving, sprinkle the perch with chopped fresh parsley. Serve the perch with artichokes and black olives hot, accompanied by side dishes of your choice.

RECIPES SIDE DISH

GRILLED VEGETABLE SALAD WITH FETA AND LEMON VINAIGRETTE

Preparation time: 20 minutes

Cooking times: 15 minutes

Doses for: 4 people

Ingredients:

2 medium courgettes, cut into slices

1 red pepper, cut into slices

1 red onion, sliced

150g feta, crumbled

For the vinaigrette:

2 tablespoons of olive oil

1 tablespoon lemon juice

1 teaspoon honey

Salt and pepper to taste

Preparation

Preheat the grill to medium heat. Lightly coat the vegetables with olive oil. Grill vegetables for 3-4 minutes per side, or until tender and lightly charred. Transfer the grilled vegetables to a bowl. In a small bowl, whisk together the olive oil, lemon juice, honey, salt, and pepper. Pour the vinaigrette over the vegetables and garnish with the feta. For a smokier flavor, you can grill vegetables on a charcoal or gas grill.

ROASTED BRUSSELS SPROUTS WITH HONEY AND SRIRACHA

Preparation time: 10 minutes

Cooking times: 25 minutes

Doses for: 4 people

Ingredients:

500 g of Brussels sprouts,

cut in half

2 tablespoons of olive oil

1 tablespoon honey

1 tablespoon sriracha

Salt and pepper to taste

Preparation

Preheat the oven to 200°C. In a large bowl, toss the Brussels sprouts with the olive oil, honey, sriracha, salt and pepper. Spread the Brussels sprouts on a baking tray lined with baking paper. Bake for 20-25 minutes, or until Brussels sprouts are tender and golden brown. If you don't have sriracha, you can substitute another type of hot sauce. Roasted Brussels sprouts can be served hot or cold.

ROASTED CARROTS WITH THYME AND PARMESAN

Preparation time: 15 minutes

Cooking times: 30 minutes

Doses for: 4 people

Ingredients:

500 g carrots, peeled

and cut into pieces

2 tablespoons of olive oil

1 teaspoon fresh thyme

Salt and pepper to taste

2 tablespoons grated parmesan

Preparation

Preheat the oven to 200°C. In a large bowl, toss the carrots with the olive oil, thyme, salt and pepper. Spread the carrots on a baking tray lined with baking paper. Bake for 20-25 minutes, or until carrots are tender and golden brown. Sprinkle with grated Parmesan before serving. Tips: For more flavor, you can add a pinch of garlic powder or onion powder to the carrots before placing them in the oven. If you like cheese, you can also add a little grated pecorino romano to the parmesan. Roasted carrots make a great side dish for chicken, fish or pork.

SAUTEED GREEN BEANS WITH GARLIC AND LEMON

Preparation time: 10 minutes

Cooking times: 10 minutes

Doses for: 4 people

Ingredients:

450 g green beans, cut

2 tablespoons of olive oil

2 cloves garlic, minced

1 tablespoon lemon juice

Salt and pepper to taste

Preparation

Heat the olive oil in a large skillet over medium-high heat. Add the garlic and cook for 30 seconds, or until fragrant. Add the green beans and cook for 5-7 minutes, or until tender. Add the lemon juice and cook for another minute. Salt and pepper to taste. Tips: For a spicier flavor, you can add a pinch of chili powder to the green beans. If you like lemon, you can add a little grated lemon zest to the green beans before serving. Sautéed green beans are a great side dish for steak, or salmon.

QUINOA SALAD WITH VEGETABLES AND FETA

Preparation time: 20 minutes

Cooking times: 15 minutes

(for the quinoa) +

cooking time for vegetables

Doses for: 4 people

Ingredients:

100 g of quinoa

200 g of feta

200 g of mixed vegetables (for example,

tomatoes, cucumbers, peppers, onions)

For the seasoning:

3 tablespoons of olive oil

1 tablespoon lemon juice

1 teaspoon dried oregano

Salt and pepper to taste

Preparation

Cook the quinoa according to the package instructions. Meanwhile, cut the vegetables into small pieces. In a large bowl, mix the cooked quinoa, vegetables and feta. For the dressing, whisk together the olive oil, lemon juice, oregano, salt and pepper. Pour the dressing over the salad and mix well. Tips: You can add other vegetables to the salad as you like. If you don't have feta, you can replace it with another type of crumbled cheese. Quinoa salad is a great dish to bring to a picnic or lunch at work.

**STEAMED VEGETABLES
WITH TAHINI SAUCE**

Preparation time: 15 minutes

Cooking times: 10-15 minutes

Doses for: 4 people

Ingredients:

500 g of mixed vegetables

(broccoli, cauliflower, carrots, green beans)

For the tahini sauce:

1/2 cup tahini

1/4 cup lemon juice

1/4 cup water

2 cloves garlic, minced

1 tablespoon olive oil

Salt and pepper to taste

Preparation

Steam the vegetables until tender. Meanwhile, prepare the tahini sauce. In a blender, blend together the tahini, lemon juice, water, garlic, olive oil, salt, and pepper until smooth. Serve the steamed vegetables with the tahini sauce on the side. Tips: You can use any kind of vegetables you like for this recipe. If the tahini sauce is too thick, you can add a little more water until you reach your desired consistency. Steamed Vegetables with Tahini Sauce is a healthy, flavorful side dish that's perfect for any meal.

ROASTED FENNEL WITH ORANGES AND OLIVES

Preparation time: 15 minutes

Cooking times: 30 minutes

Doses for: 4 people

Ingredients:

3 medium fennels, cut into wedges

1 orange, cut into slices

1/2 cup pitted black olives

2 tablespoons of olive oil

1 tablespoon lemon juice

1 teaspoon dried oregano

Salt and pepper to taste

Preparation

Preheat the oven to 200°C. In a large bowl, mix the fennel, oranges, olives, olive oil, lemon juice, oregano, salt and pepper. Spread the mixture onto a baking tray lined with baking paper. Bake for 20-25 minutes, or until the fennel is tender and lightly browned. Tips: You can add other ingredients to this recipe, such as onions, peppers or tomatoes. If you like a stronger flavor, you can marinate the fennel in olive oil, lemon juice, herbs and spices for 30 minutes before cooking. Roasted fennel with oranges and olives is a great side dish for chicken, fish or pork.

GRILLED AUBERGINES WITH TOMATOES AND MOZZARELLA

Preparation time: 20 minutes

Cooking times: 20 minutes

Doses for: 4 people

Ingredients:

2 medium aubergines, cut into slices

2 tomatoes, cut into slices

1 mozzarella, cut into slices

2 tablespoons of olive oil

1 tablespoon chopped fresh basil

Salt and pepper to taste

Preparation

Heat a grill over medium-high heat. Brush the aubergines with olive oil and grill for 5-7 minutes per side, or until tender and with grill marks. Arrange the grilled aubergines on a serving plate. Add the tomatoes, mozzarella and basil. Drizzle with remaining olive oil, salt and pepper to taste. Tips: You can add other ingredients to this recipe, such as grilled onions, peppers or mushrooms. If you like cheese, you can add some grated parmesan to the mozzarella. Grilled aubergines with tomatoes and mozzarella are a great appetizer or side dish.

SAUTÉED SPINACH WITH GARLIC AND CHILI

Preparation time: 10 minutes

Cooking times: 5 minutes

Doses for: 4 people

Ingredients:

450 g of fresh spinach

2 tablespoons of olive oil

2 cloves garlic, minced

1/2 red chili pepper, chopped (optional)

Salt and pepper to taste

Preparation

Wash the spinach carefully and drain well. Heat the olive oil in a large skillet over medium heat. Add the garlic and chili pepper (if using) and cook for 30 seconds, or until fragrant. Add the spinach and cook for 2-3 minutes, or until wilted. Salt and pepper to taste. Tips: You can add other ingredients to this recipe, such as onions, tomatoes or mushrooms. If you like spicier flavor, you can add more crushed red pepper. Sauteed spinach with garlic and chili peppers is a great side dish for chicken, fish or tofu.

STUFFED MUSHROOMS

Preparation time: 20 minutes

Cooking times: 25 minutes

Doses for: 4 people

Ingredients:

400 g large button mushrooms

1/2 onion, chopped

1 clove garlic, minced

100 g of breadcrumbs

50 g of butter

2 tablespoons of parsley

fresh chopped

Salt and pepper to taste

Preparation

Preheat the oven to 180°C. Wash the mushrooms and remove the stems. In a large skillet, melt the butter over medium heat. Add the onion and garlic and cook for 5 minutes, or until tender. Add the breadcrumbs, parsley, salt and pepper and cook for another minute. Fill the mushrooms with the breadcrumb mixture. Arrange the stuffed mushrooms on a baking tray lined with baking paper. Bake for 20-25 minutes, or until mushrooms are tender and golden. Tips: You can add other ingredients to the filling, such as grated cheese, cooked ham cubes or chopped vegetables. If you like more flavor, you can brush the mushrooms with a little olive oil before cooking them. Stuffed mushrooms are a great side dish.

CONCLUSION

Thank you for joining us on your journey through "Super Metabolism Diet 2025". I hope this book has inspired and guided you towards a healthier and more vital life. Now that you have acquired valuable knowledge about how your metabolism works and strategies to optimize it, I invite you to put what you have learned into practice. Let your success become an inspiration to others. I kindly ask you to share your experience by leaving a review. Thank you very much to all the readers for their support and commitment in pursuing well-being. Thank you for embarking on this journey with me through the pages of the "Super Metabolism Diet 2025". During our journey, we explored the depths of metabolism, discovering its secrets and learning how we can harness its potential to improve our overall health and well-being. Now, as we reach the conclusion of this book, I want to express my gratitude to you, dear reader. Thank you for dedicating your time and attention to these pages, for showing a sincere interest in understanding and improving your health. I hope the information and strategies shared here have inspired and motivated you towards positive change in your life. Whether you've started this journey to lose weight, increase energy, or improve your overall health, I hope you've found what you're looking for and are ready to put what you've learned into practice. I kindly ask you to take a moment to share your experience reading this book by leaving an honest review. Your words can help other readers discover and benefit from this book, and for that I will be eternally grateful. Finally, I would like to thank all the readers who made the creation of this book possible. Your support and commitment to pursuing health and wellness is a constant source of inspiration. May you continue your journey to a healthier and happier life with confidence and determination. May you find joy, satisfaction and success every step of the way. Thanks again for accompanying me on this journey. May your path be illuminated by the light of continued health and happiness. With infinite gratitude,

[KLARLOCK]

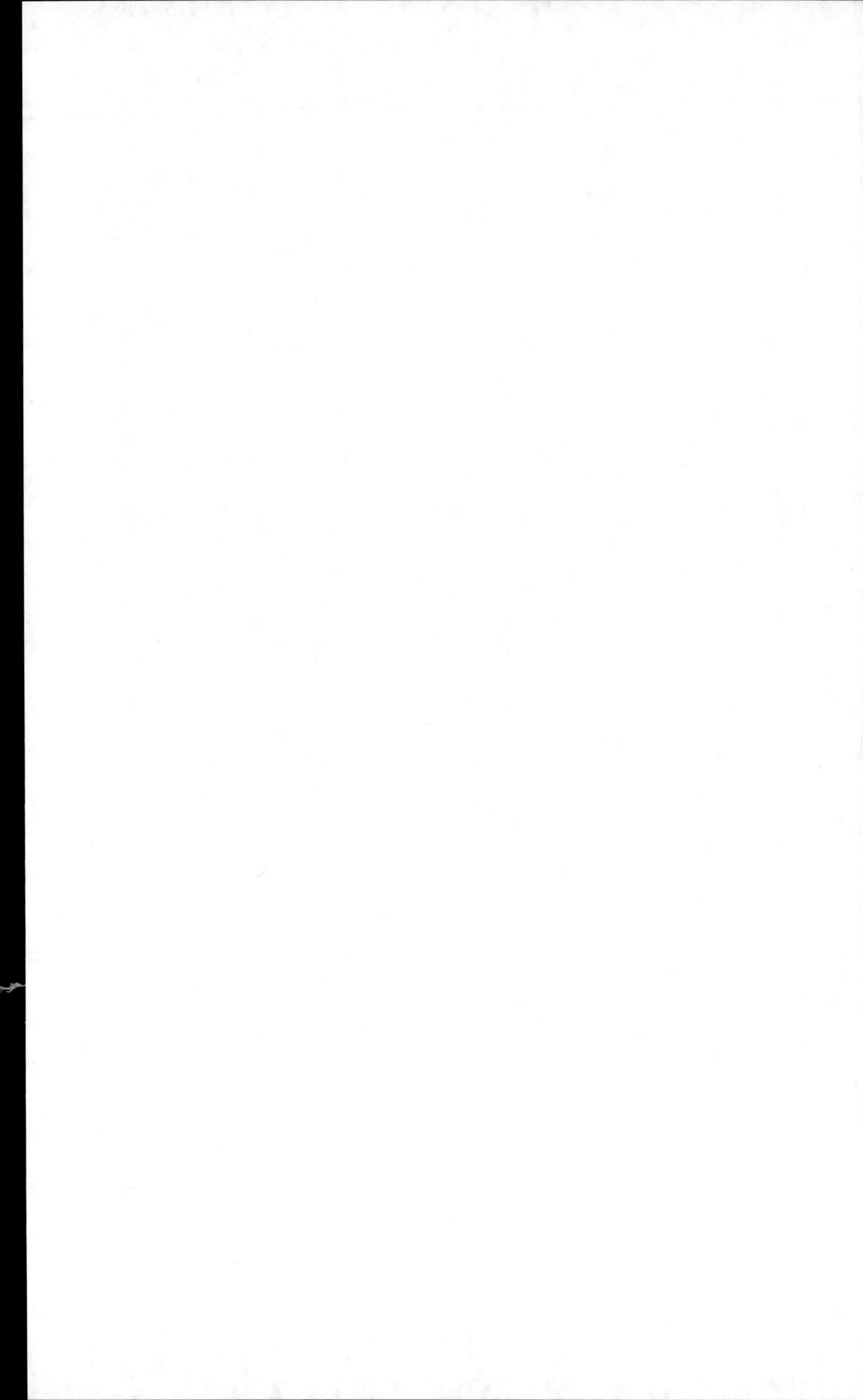